AF540435

Animal Genetics and Breeding
Animal Nutrition
Livestock Production and Management

www.nipaers.com

Browse, Search, Read & Buy...

Print Books eChapters
eBooks Publishers
Forthcoming Subject Catalogues
New Titles

Online Resources on:

- ✓ Current Affairs
- ✓ Reasoning, Logic & Aptitude
- ✓ Competitive Examinations
- ✓ English Language Lab
- ✓ Writing & Pronunciation Tools
- ✓ Personality Development
- ✓ Online Programmes for Professionals
- ✓ Interview Preparation

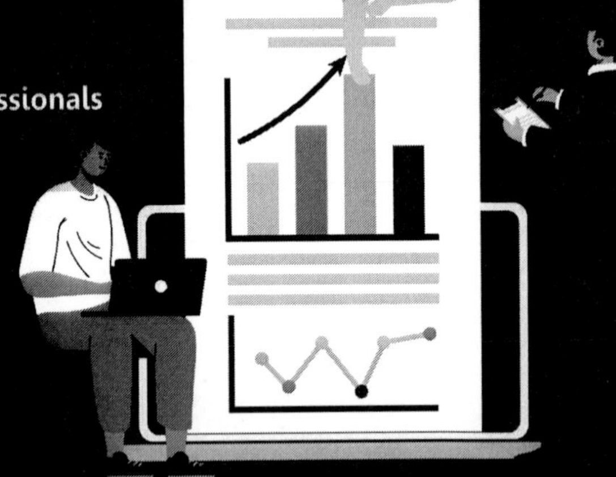

Pay Using

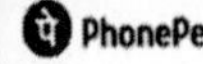

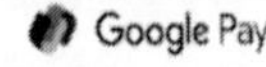

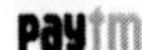

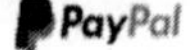

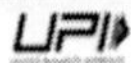

CC Avenue

Animal Genetics and Breeding
Animal Nutrition
Livestock Production and Management

Narendra Singh Jadon, M.V.Sc., Ph.D.
Professor and Head, Department of Surgery and Radiology
College of Veterinary and Animal Sciences
G.B. Pant University of Agriculture and Technology
Pantnagar, Udham Singh Nagar, Uttarakhand – 263 145

Brijesh Singh, M.Sc. (Ag.), Ph.D.
Professor, Department of Livestock Production Management
College of Veterinary and Animal Sciences
G.B. Pant University of Agriculture and Technology
Pantnagar, Udham Singh Nagar, Uttarakhand – 263 145

Nikhil Pratap Singh, B.Sc. Ag., PGDMA (NAARM)
Research Scholar, Venketashwara University
Gajraula-244 221, Uttar Pradesh

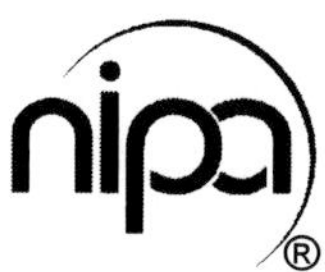

NEW INDIA PUBLISHING AGENCY
Pitam Pura, New Delhi – 110 088

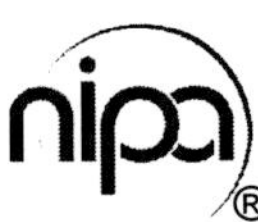

NEW INDIA PUBLISHING AGENCY
101, Vikas Surya Plaza, CU Block, LSC Market
Pitam Pura, New Delhi 110 034, India
Phone: +91 (11)27 34 17 17 Fax: +91(11) 27 34 16 16
Email: info@nipabooks.com
Web: www.nipabooks.com

Feedback at feedbacks@nipabooks.com

© 2018 Authors

ISBN: 978-9387973-27-5

All rights reserved, no part of this publication may be reproduced, stored in a retrieval system or transmitted in any form or by any means, electronic, mechanical, photocopying, recording or otherwise without the prior written permission of the publisher or the copyright holder.

This book contains information obtained from authentic and highly regarded sources. Reasonable efforts have been made to publish reliable data and information, but the author/s, editor/s and publisher cannot assume responsibility for the validity of all materials or the consequences of their use. The author/s, editor/s and publisher have attempted to trace and acknowledge the copyright holders of all material reproduced in this publication and apologize to copyright holders if permission and acknowledgements to publish in this form have not been taken. If any copyright material has not been acknowledged please write and let us know so we may rectify it, in subsequent reprints.

Trademark notice: Presentations, logos (the way they are written/presented) in this book are under the trademarks of the publisher and hence, if copied/resembled the copier will be prosecuted under the law.

Composed and Designed by NIPA

Preface

I felt the need of a suitable objective type book on animal genetics and breeding, nutrition, and livestock production and management to meet the requirement of the undergraduate students. Presently, I also feel the necessity not less than I find the students getting lost time in larger volumes of books on different aspects. This inspired me to write multiple choice books on the subjects specially meant for the students of B.V.Sc. & A.H., civil services aspirants and general educationists. This book deals comprehensively in all important aspects of animal genetics and breeding, nutrition and livestock management. In this book I don't pretend to claim credit for any original contribution on the subject rather than it should be viewed as a concise collection of various important topics. This book has been divided into 3 sections dealing with animal genetics and breeding, animal nutrition, livestock production and management, respectively.

I am indebted to Dr. Deepti Bodh, Assistant professor in department of Veterinary Surgery and Radiology for her generous and sincere help and advice while writing this book. My thanks are also due to one of my graduating student Dr. Ramanpreet Singh Sandhu for the support rendered by him. The contribution of the co-authors of the book is duly acknowledged.

I shall be failing in my duties if I don't mention the name of my teacher Dr. Amresh Kumar, former Vice-Chancellor of G.B. Pant University of Agri. & Tech., Pantnagar without whose encouragement this work could have not been possible.

I am grateful to my wife, Mrs. Sudha Singh for the strain she has tolerated so patiently and the load she took off my shoulders-responsibilities that could have diverted my attention from the academic endeavors.

I am fully confident that the reader would show lot of interest in this book specially the undergraduate and post graduate students of veterinary colleges across the country, teachers, researchers, trainers, civil service aspirants and general educationists.

Any suggestions for the improvement of the book will be thankfully received.

Narendra S. Jadon

Contents

1

Animal Genetics and Breeding Biostatistics

Q.1. True and False

1. True — The data generated by processing the original data is called secondary data.

2. False — Median and mode can undergo algebric manipulations like arithmetic mean.

3. True — RBD is more accurate than CRD for most types of experimental work.

4. True — Coefficient of variation may be utilized for comparing two data of different units.

5. True — Frequency polygon is made by joining the middle points of tops of each rectangle of histogram.

6. True — Mean sum of squares are the variances.

7. False — Percentile is a measure of kurtosis.

8. True — At an ordinate $x = m$ in normal curve, the mean = mode = median.

9. False — Goodness of fit is tested by t-test.

10. True — Any two events A and B are said to be independent if P(AB)=P(A). P(B).

11. True — In a test of significance if a null hypothesis is rejected at 5% level it will also be rejected at 1% level of significance.

12. True Skewness is the measure of asymmetry of distribution.

13. True Pie diagram is a circular diagram.

14. True The mean and mode are always equal in case of normal distribution.

15. False Histogram and frequency polygon are same.

16. True Egg production in poultry is an example of discontinuous variable.

17. True The standard error is equal to standard deviation divided by the square root of number of observations.

18. True RBD is inappropriate when experimental units are heterogenous.

19. True Mean and mode are expressed in same unit.

20. False Quartile range is a measure of central tendency.

21. False Regression coefficient lies between -1 and +1.

22. False LD 50 and ED 50 are same.

23. True In Poisson distribution the mean and variance are same.

24. True Correlation coefficient range between -1 and +1.

25. True For two samples, the square root of F has student's t distribution.

26. True Range is a measure of dispersion.

27. False Variance is a measure of central tendency.

28. True Accepting the null hypothesis, when it is false, is called type-II error.

29. False The number 111 are read as one hundred and eleven.

30. True In the number 1010 each 1 has the same weightage.

31. True String variables are non-numeric variable.

32. True Pie diagram is used to depict the proportions of the different classes.

33. True The product of regression of y on x (byx) and regression of x on y (bxy) is always positive.

34. True Paired t-test is applied when the two samples are dependent.

35. True Chi-square test is used to study the goodness of fit between the observed and expected ratios.

36. True DNA is found in mitochondria also.

37. False In poultry the male is heterogametic sex.

38. False The linked genes follow the Mendel's law of independent assortment.

39. False In Klinefelter's syndrome, two barr bodies are present.

40. True Error mean square is equal to within group mean squares.

41. False Sum of squares of observations is always less than squares of total sum of observations.

42. True The square root of variance of a population is equal to standard error of sample mean.

43. True Sample size for estimation of mean can not be known in advance.

44. False Mean ± 2 s.d. covers approximately 90 percent area under normal curve.

45. False Geometric mean is most appropriate average when emphasis is on the amount of change rather than rate of change.

46. True Coefficient of variation is a measure of dispersion.

47. True Shift of origin has no effect on the correlation coefficient.

48. True In parallel line assay the average response to drug is linearly related to the log of the dose.

49. False Milk yield is an example of discontinuous variable.

50. True Sum of deviations from the mean is equal to zero.

51. False Range is the measure of central tendency.

52. True Coefficient of correlation is independent of change of origin.

53. False Regression coefficient of Y on X and X on Y are always equal.

54. True Standard deviation is a measure of dispersion.

55. False CRD can be used where experimental material is heterogenous.

56. True Coefficient of variation carries no unit.

57. False Histogram is used to depict the frequencies of the discrete classes.

58. False The two cumulative frequency curves, greater than type and less than type intersect each other at mean.

59. True Correlation has no unit.

60. True Variance is independent of origin.

61. True Arithmetic mean is the best measure of central tendency.

62. False The theory of pangenesis was proposed by Weismann.

63. False During crossing over there is exchange of chromosomal segments between sister chromatids of a chromosome.

64. True Arithmetic mean is most appropriate average when emphasis is on the amount of change rather than rate of change.

65. False In normal distribution, mean and mode coincide but not median.

66. True Mean and variance are not equal for binomial distribution.

67. False Mean±SE2 includes 95.45 percent area of the normal curve.

68. False Kurtosis measures the degree of asymmetry of a curve.

69. False In binomial distribution mean and variance are equal.

70. False The mean of data will not change when a constant is subtracted from each observation.

71. True Median is most accurate measure of central tendency for a data containing extreme values.

72. True Sample means from a normal distributed population will also be normally distributed.

73. True Probit analysis is useful in quantal response.

74. False Type–I error is more serious than type-II error.

75. True Diagrammatic representation of data can be used for comparative studies.

76. False A bimodal frequency curve has three maxima.

77. True Mode is not usually affected by extreme values.

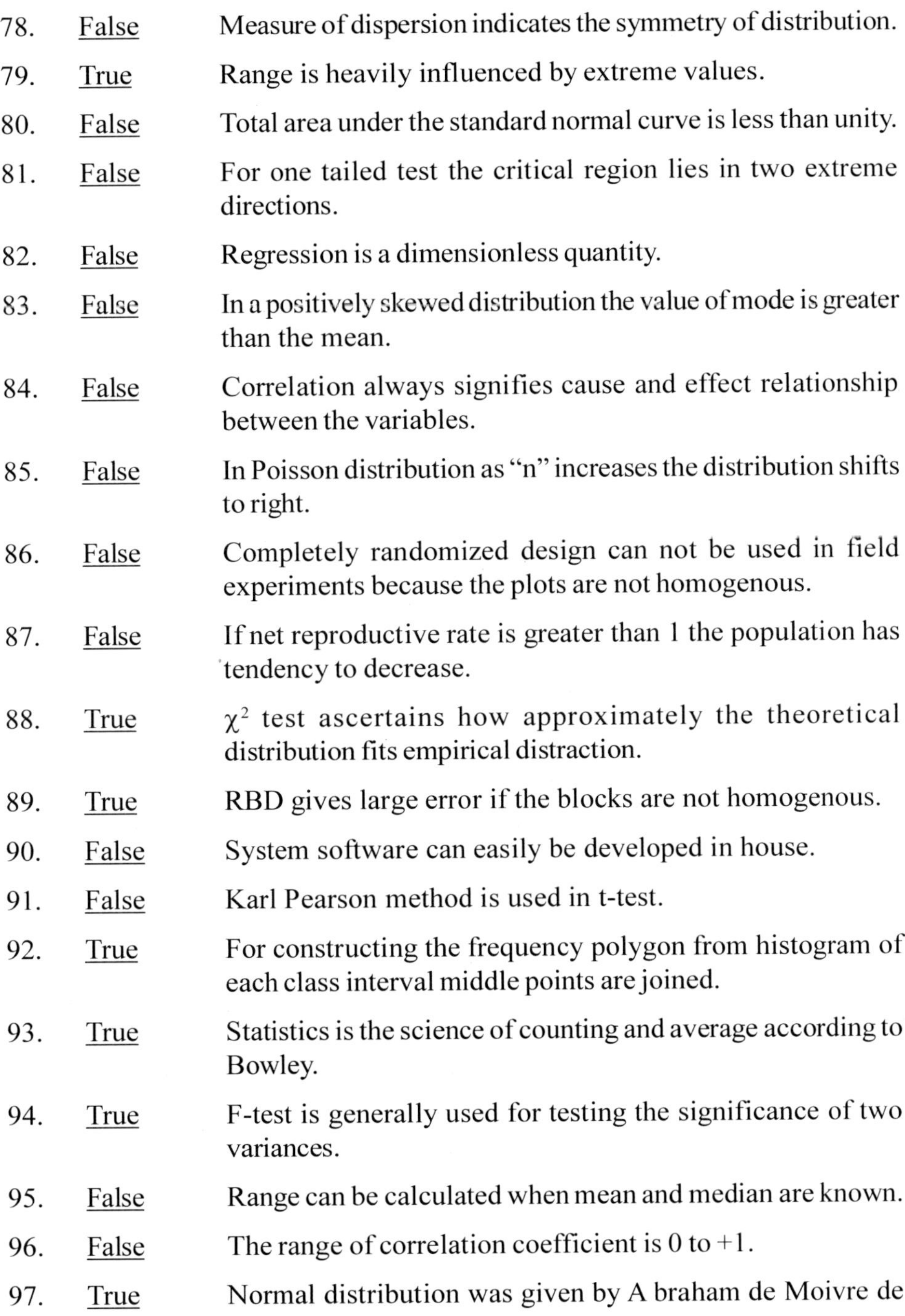

78. False Measure of dispersion indicates the symmetry of distribution.

79. True Range is heavily influenced by extreme values.

80. False Total area under the standard normal curve is less than unity.

81. False For one tailed test the critical region lies in two extreme directions.

82. False Regression is a dimensionless quantity.

83. False In a positively skewed distribution the value of mode is greater than the mean.

84. False Correlation always signifies cause and effect relationship between the variables.

85. False In Poisson distribution as "n" increases the distribution shifts to right.

86. False Completely randomized design can not be used in field experiments because the plots are not homogenous.

87. False If net reproductive rate is greater than 1 the population has tendency to decrease.

88. True χ^2 test ascertains how approximately the theoretical distribution fits empirical distraction.

89. True RBD gives large error if the blocks are not homogenous.

90. False System software can easily be developed in house.

91. False Karl Pearson method is used in t-test.

92. True For constructing the frequency polygon from histogram of each class interval middle points are joined.

93. True Statistics is the science of counting and average according to Bowley.

94. True F-test is generally used for testing the significance of two variances.

95. False Range can be calculated when mean and median are known.

96. False The range of correlation coefficient is 0 to +1.

97. True Normal distribution was given by A braham de Moivre de Moivre.

98. False Standard deviation is not the best measure of dispersion in which all observations participate.

99. False — Mode is the best measure of central tendency.

100. False — Rejecting a null hypothesis (H_0) when it is true is called type-II error.

101. True — Level of significance (a) is the probability of committing type-I error.

102. True — The value 7.0 E_4 is valid integer constant.

Q.2 Multiple Choice Questions

1. The regression equation of Y on X can be written as:

   a. y^ = y¯+bx b. y^ = y¯(bx)

   c. y^ = y¯bx d. y^ = y¯/bx

2. The variance may be defined as:

   a. Mean squared deviation from mean

   b. Mean deviation from mean

   c. Deviation from range

   d. Square root of standard deviation

3. Which is true for a correlation coefficient:

   a. It has a unit b. Varies from 0 to 1

   c. Varies from-1to+1 d. Always meaningful mean

4. The range of regression coefficient is:

   a. -1 to 0 b. -1 to +1

   c. - ∝ to + ∝ d. 1 to 1000

5. The normal curve is also known as:

   a. Leptokurtic b. Mesokurtic

   c. Platykuritic d. None of the above

6. Which of the following is square root of variance:

   a. Standard deviation b. Mean deviation

   c. Range d. Both a & b

7. Standard error of sample may be determined by following formula:

a. SD/√ n | **b. SD/ √ n-1**
c. SD* √ n | d. AD/mean * √ n

8. Karl Pearson measure is used:

a. For measuring kurtosis | **b. For measuring skewness**
c. Both a & b | d. For measuring correlation

9. The chances of throwing at least one ace in a single throw with two dice are:

a. 5/36 | **b. 11/36**
c. 1/36 | d. 4/36

10. Primary data are:

a. Raw, original and unprocessed data
b. Based on choice of enumerator
c. Statistical manipulation
d. Obtained from data base

11. Critical difference test is used to:

a. Compare subclass means
b. Compare two variances
c. Compare one mean of one effect and the other mean of other effect
d. It is done after chi-square test

12. The two lines of regression are same at:

a. r = 0.5 | b. r = 0.0
c. r = 0.89 | **d. r = ± 1**

13. Which of the following biological process follows the law of probability:

a. Gamete formation | b. Hormone secretion
c. Metabolic process | d. Metamorphosis

14. Student t-test was discovered by:

    a. Bernoulli b. Galton
    c. W.S.Gosset d. D.B.Duncan

15. The F-value is:

    a. Estimate error variance **b. Variance ratio**
    c. Mean difference d. Ratio of means

16. Which of the following can not be calculated if the data series has a negative value:

    a. Arithmetic mean b. Median
    c. Mode **d. Geometric mean**

17. The population in which supply of members is never exhausted by any sampling process:

    a. Finite population **b. Infinite population**
    c. Real population d. Hypothetical population

18. The repetition of the treatments under investigation is known as:

    a. Randomization b. Local control
    c. Replication d. None of the above

19. The experimental design which simultaneously controls the variation in two directions is known as:

    a. RBD b. CRD
    c. LSD d. None of the above

20. Which one of the following is not type of average:

    a. Arithmetic mean b. Geometric mean
    c. Harmonic mean **d. Median**

21. Parameters of binomial distribution are:

    a. n and p b. p and q
    c. np and npq d. None of the above

22. Accepting a true hypothesis is:

    a. Type-l error b. Type-II error
    c. Any of a and b **d. None of the above**

23. Mean deviation is a measure of:
    a. Central tendency
    b. Dispersion
    c. Skewness
    d. All of the above
24. To test sample mean with the population mean we use:
    a. f-test
    b. t-test
    c. Chi square test
    d. None of the above
25. In normal distribution :
    a. Mean and median are same but mode is different
    b. Mean and mode are same but median is different
    c. Mean and mode are same but mean is different
    d. Mean, median and mode are same
26. The mean and variance are same for :
    a. Normal distribution
    b. Binominal distribution
    c. Poisson distribution
    d. Chi-square distribution
27. Central moments are calculated from:
    a. Mean
    b. Median
    c. Mode
    d. None of the above
28. Median is equivalent to:
    a. Fist quartile
    b. Second quartile
    c. Third quartile
    d. None of the above
29. Regression coefficient is:
    a. Unit free
    b. Unit as correlation coefficient
    c. Same unit as mean
    d. None of the above
30. RBD is simplest design where:
    a. All basic principles of design are used
    b. Only replication is used

c. Replication and randomization is used

d. No principle is used

31. In simple random sampling:

a. With and without replacement samplings are same

b. With replacement sampling is more efficient than without replacement

c. Without replacement sampling is more efficient than with replacement sampling

d. None of the above

32. Effective dose for 50% killing is:

a. LD-50 **b. ED-50**

c. Both LD-50 and ED-50 d. None of the above

33. Critical values of Z for two tailed test at 0.05 level of significance is:

a. -1.96 and 1.96 b. -2.81 and 2.81

c. -2.58 and 2.58 d. None of the above

34. Geometric mean is:

a. Greater than arithmetic mean

b. Less than harmonic mean

c. Both a & b

d. None of the above

35. The standard deviation of a mean is often called:

a. Standard error b. Variance of mean

c. Mean square d. None of the above

36. The LSD uses the pooled error variance is basically:

a. One tailed f-test **b. Student's t-test**

c. Chi-square test of homogeneity d. None of the above

37. Probability of getting 2 in single throw of a fair dice is:

a. 2/6 **b. 1/6**

c. 1 d. 3/6

38. Correlation coefficient is:

a. Always positive
b. Always negative
c. Either positive or negative
d. None of the above

39. The graphic outputs are performed over text output because:

a. It is easier to generate graphic output than text.
b. Graphic is produced in multicolor and text is in black and white
c. Graphics are condensed and quickly understandable
d. It always takes longer time to generate text

40. The regression coefficient between two variables is independent of :

a. Origin
b. Scale
c. Both a & b
d. None of the above

41. If the regression of y on x is negative, the regression of x on y will be:

a. Positive
b. Negative
c. Either positive or negative
d. Zero

42. The measure of central tendency affected by the extreme values is:

a. Arithmetic mean
b. Mode
c. Median
d. Both b & c

43. The normal curve is:

a. Symmetrical
b. Positively skewed
c. Negatively skewed
d. Bimodal

44. For comparing two samples, with different means, for their variability the best measure is:

a. Variance
b. Standard deviation
c. Co-efficient of variation
d. All of the above

45. In completely randomized design (CRD) the data is classified:

a. One way
b. Two way
c. Three way
d. More than three way

46. For testing the association between incidence of peptic ulcers and ABO blood group system we can apply:

a. T test b. F test

c. Z test **d. Chi square test**

47. In two tailed test the alternative hypothesis is:

a. $m_1 > m_2$ b. $m_1 = m_2$

c. $m_1 < m_2$ **d.** $\mathbf{m_1{}^1m_2}$

48. The appropriate test for testing of significance for qualitative data:

a. T-test b. Z-test

c. F-test **d. Chi-square test**

49. Multiple mean comparisons are done by:

a. LSD b. T-test

c. DMRT d. None of the above

50. When the dose-response relationship does not lead to parallel lines we can use:

a. Parallel line assay **b. Slope ratio assay**

c. Both of the above d. None of the above

51. Confidence interval for ratio of variances can be calculated using:

a. Z-distribution b. T-distribution

c. Chi-square distribution **d. None of the above**

52. Correlation and regression coefficients are equal if:

a. Covarinces are less than zero

b. Covarinces are more than zero

c. Variances are equal

d. Variances is unity

53. The number of possible combinations to form a group of 6 patients out of 10 patients:

a. 151200 b. 5040

c. 210 d. 222

54. The term gene was coined by:

a. Wilhelm Johannsen
b. George Mendel
c. Hardy-Weinberg
d. Lush

55. dBASE, word star, word perfect, and page maker are:

a. System software
b. Application software
c. High level programming languages
d. Low level programming languages

56. Best estimate of central tendency in normal distribution is:

a. Geometric mean
b. Arithmetic mean
c. Harmonic mean
d. None of the above

57. Frequency distribution can be represented graphically by:

a. Pie diagram
b. Bar diagram
c. Multiple bar diagram
d. Ogive

58. The point of intersection of the less than and greater than ogive corresponds to:

a. Mean
b. Median
c. Geometric mean
d. None of the above

59. Which test of significance is used to testing independence of attributes:

a. Chi-square test
b. T-test
c. Z-test
d. F-test

60. The level of significance indicates:

a. Power of test
b. Probability of committing type I error
c. Probability of committing type II error
d. None of the above

61. For one way ANOVA with k treatments and n observations in all, the number of degree of freedom for numerator is:

a. K-1
b. n-k
c. n-1
d. None of the above

62. Sex linked alleles cannot be passed from a :

a. Woman to her daughters

b. Man to his grandsons

c. Man to his sons

d. Woman to her grand daughters

63. To test a sample mean with the population mean we use:

a. t-test b. F test

c. Chi square test d. None of the above

64. Litter size and average birth weight is example of:

a. Positive correlation **b. Negative correlation**

c. No correlation d. All of the above

65. Median is a measure of:

a. Central tendency b. Dispersion

c. Skewness d. All of the above

66. Basic principle of design of experiments is:

a. Replication b. Randomization

c. Local control **d. All of the above**

67. The correlation coefficient between two variables is independent of:

a. Origin b. Scale

c. Both of the above d. None of the above

68. The different types of software include:

a. System b. Service

c. Application **d. All of the above**

69. The measure of central tendency not affected by the extreme values is:

a. Arithmetic mean b. Geometric mean

c. Harmonic mean **d. Median**

70. In randomized block design (RBD) the data is classified:

a. One way **b. Two way**

c. Three way d. More than there way

73. For testing the association between incidence of Malaria and ABO blood group system we can apply:

    a. T test b. F test
    c. Z test **d. Chi-square test**

74. In one tailed test the alternative hypothesis is:

    a. ml > m2 b. ml = m2
    c. ml < m2 **d. a or c**

75. The mean of Poisson distribution is:

    a. Greater than its variance b. Less than its variance
    c. Equal to its variance d. None of the above

76. Standard error of sample mean depends on:

    a. Number of observations b. Variability in the data
    c. Both of the above d. None of the above

77. Total area under standard normal curve is:

    a. Greater than one b. Less than one
    c. Equal to one d. None of the above

78. Which test of significance is used to test independence of attributes:

    a. Chi-square test b. T test
    c. Z test d. F test

79. The level of significance indicates:

    a. Power of test
    b. Probability of committing type-I error
    c. Probability of committing type-II error
    d. None of the above

80. Methods of studying correlation are:

    a. Scatter diagram b. Graphical method
    c. Coefficient of correlation **d. All of the above**

81. The most appropriate measure of dispersion for data measured in different units is:

a. Range b. Variance

c. Coefficient of variation d. Standard deviation

82. In Poisson distribution the mean is equal to:

a. Variance b. Twice the variance

c. Half of variance d. Standard deviation

83. Standard normal distribution has mean equal to:

a. One b. Two

c. Zero d. None of the above

84. To know the difference between two sample means the most appropriate test would be:

a. Z-test b. T-test

c. F test **d. None of the above**

85. The sign of correlation coefficient depend upon:

a. Sign of covariance b. Magnitude of covariance

c. Magnitude of variances d. None of the above

86. The student distribution was given by:

a. Karl Pearson b. Snedecor

c. W.S. Gosset d. R.A. Fisher

87. If 15 is subtracted from each observation the standard deviation of data will be:

a. Increased by 15 b. Decreased by 15

c. Increased by 25 **d. Same**

88. The arithmetic, geometric and harmonic means will be equal if:

a. All numbers are identical b. All numbers are different

c. Both of the above d. None of the above

89. Standard deviation of the mean is called:

a. Standard error of mean b. Variance

c. Both of the above d. None of the above

90. Total area under the normal curve is:

a. 2 **b. 1**

c. 0 d. None of the above

91. In binominal and Poisson distribution the variable is:

a. Continuous **b. Discrete**

c. Semi-continuous d. None of the above

92. Mean and variance will be equal in the data following:

a. Binominal distribution **b. Poisson distribution**

c. Normal distribution d. Chi-square distribution

93. The following test of significance is applied to quantitative data:

a. Z-test b. T-test

c. F-test **d. All of the above**

94. Covariance a measure of the joint variation of two variables may be:

a. Positive b. Negative

c. Either positive or negative d. None of the above

95. One of the methods of determining mode is:

a. 2 median – 3 mean b. 3 median + 2 mean

c. 3 median – 2 mean d. 2 median + 3 mean

97. Which of the following is not a genetic component of variance:

a. V_A b. V_D

c. V_E d. V_I

98. Variance is expressed as deviation from:

a. Mode b. Median

c. Mean d. Variable

99. ANOVA is used for:

a. Estimation of h^2 b. Estimation of correlation

c. Analysis of covariance **d. Analysis of variance**

100. Which of the following type of error is used for rejecting a null hypothesis (Ho) when it is true:

a. **Type-I error** b. Type-II error

c. Both a & b d. None of the above

101. Relative measure of dispersion is:

a. Mean deviation b. Standard deviation

c. Both a & b **d. Coefficient of variation**

102. Coefficient of correlation was introduced by:

a. Karl Pearson b. Peterson

c. Karl Correns d. Karl Peterson

103. The significance of two small sample means is tested by the:

a. Z-test b. F-test

c. t-test d. All of the above

104. In statistics we deal with:

a. Single observation b. Two observations

c. Many observations d. All of the above

105. The measure of the central tendency in which all the observations are included, is:

a. Arithmetic mean b. Harmonic mean

c. Geometric mean **d. All of the above**

106. The standard deviation of 4, 4, 4 and 4 shall be:

a. 0 b. 4

c. 8 d. 16

107. Student's' distribution was discovered by:

a. Karl Pearson b. R.A.Fisher

c. F.Yates **d. William Gosset**

108. Test of significance includes:

a. 't' test b. χ^2 test

c. 'F' test **d. All of the above**

109. Which average is very much affected by extreme observations:

a. Mode b. Median

c. Arithmetic mean d. None of the above

110. Measure of dispersion includes:

a. Standard deviation b. Mean deviation

c. Range **d. All of the above**

111. Chi-square test is a:

a. Measure of central tendency b. Measure of dispersion

c. Measure of correlation **d. Test of goodness of fit**

112. The word statistics is used to refer the techniques and methods used in the :

a. Collection of data b. Analysis of data

c. Interpretation of data **d. All of the above**

113. If the number of values is even, then the median is :

a. Average of two middle values b. Middle value

c. Both a & b d. None of the above

Q.3. Fill in the Blanks

1. P(AB)=P(A). P(B/A)=P (B). P(A/B) is the theorem of ***compound probability.***
2. The full expression of LD50 is ***lethal dose 50.***
3. Measures of dispersion are ***range variance and SD/SE.***
4. The formula for co efficient of variation is $\frac{SD}{mean}$ *X 100.*
5. For making pie diagram the data is converted into ***percentage.***
6. The co efficient of skewness = ***mean- mode/SD.*** / ***standard*** ***deviation***
7. The formula for determining the standard error of sample is ***SDÖ n-1.***
8. The suitable measure of central tendency for deciding the wages is ***median.***
9. When all the observations are arranged in ascending or descending order of magnitude the middle one is known as ***median.***
10. To test the equality of two sample means ***t-test*** is used.

11. ***Mode*** is a variable which occurs most frequently when several samples are drawn from a population.

12. When the events are such that occurrence one is incompatible with the occurrence of any of the others, they are known as ***mutually exclusive*** events.

13. The process of selecting individual from a population is known as ***sampling.***

14. Sample surveys deal with samples drawn from population which contain a finite number of units known as ***F-test.***

15. If there is no relationship between the variables, they are said to be ***uncorrelated/ independent.***

16. ***Analysis of variance*** is a simple arithmetical process of sorting out the components of variation in a given data.

17. The mean of a sample will be increased by ***5,*** if 5 is added to each observation.

18. The skewness of a symmetric distribution is ***zero.***

19. Mortality is defined as ratio of number of deaths and ***mid point population.***

20. Fertility rate is number of birth per ***1000 female in child bearing age*** in thc population.

21. Correlation coefficient measures the degree of linear relationship between ***two*** variables.

22. ANOVA is a method to split total ***variation*** in the data to assignable causes.

23. In t-test, the two population's variances are assumed to be ***equal.***

24. The unit of mean and SD are ***same.***

25. ***Skewness*** is the degree of asymmetry of a distribution.

26. Bar diagram represent only ***quantitative*** variable.

27. The sum of deviations of a set of observations from their mean is ***zero.***

28. Probability of getting a male calf in a single calving is ***50*** percent.

29. When experimental units are homogeneous ***CRD*** design is appropriate.

30. In practice a level of significance of ***0.05 or 0.01*** is customary.

31. In the probability of occurrence of an event is 0.4 and another independent even is 0.2, the probability of their simultaneous occurrence will be ***0.08.***

32. In negatively skewed curve the median lies to the ***Left*** of the mode.

33. The inequality of variances between two samples can be tested by ***f-test.***

34. In ***CRD*** design the experimental units should be homogeneous.

35. The three basic principles of an experimental design are ***replication, randomization and local control.***

36. ***C.V.*** is used for comparing the variability of two traits measured in different units.

37. The correlation coefficient between two dependent variables range from ***1 to +1.***

38. **RBD** design is appropriate when the experimental units are homogeneous.

39. In ANOVA experimental errors are assumed to be normally and independently distributed with mean ***zero*** and ***constant*** variance.

40. In parallel line assay the average response to drug is linearly related to the ***log*** of dose.

41. Binomial distribution tends to approach Poisson distribution when sample size is ***large*** and probability of success is ***small.***

42. As the number of observations increases the t-distribution tends to approach ***Z-distribution.***

43. Experimental errors under ANOVA have mean ***zero*** and constant variances.

44. LD_{50} stands for ***median lethal dose.***

45. When the experimental units are heterogeneous ***randomized block*** design is appropriate.

46. Kurtosis indicates ***peakedness*** of the curve.

47. Probability of two male calves in two calving is ***¼.***

48. ***Normal*** distribution is continuous probability distribution.

49. For a given data ***harmonic*** mean is equal or less than geometric mean.

50. The limit of probability is ***0-1.***

51. The mode is the measure of ***central tendency.***

52. The relation between coefficient of correlation and regression coefficient is ***r=byx × bxy.***

53. Milk production and fat percent in milk is an example of ***negative*** correlation.

54. When experimental material is homogenous we use ***simple random*** sampling.

55. In histogram ***classes*** are taken on X axis.

56. The sum of deviations of all the observations from the arithmetic mean is equal to ***zero***.

57. In a perfectly symmetrical curve the third moment is equal to ***zero.***

58. If the probability of occurrence of an event is 0.5 and another independent event is 0.25 the probability of their simultaneous occurrence will be ***0.125.***

59. In positively skewed curve the median lies to the ***right*** of the mode.

60. ***Paired t-test*** is used to compare two treatment means if the experimental units are dependent.

61. A test commonly used to measure goodness of fit is ***Chi-square test***.

62. Variance is ***square*** of standard deviation.

63. Poisson distribution is a ***discrete*** probability distribution.

64. ***Coefficient of variation*** is used to compare the variability in two characters measured in different units.

65. Class interval in frequency distribution can be decided with the help of ***Sturge's*** rule.

66. Rejecting a null hypothesis when it is true is called ***type-I*** error.

67. The CRD is used only when the experimental units are ***homogeneous.***

68. 'F' test is used to test equality of ***variance.***

69. ***Skewness*** deals with direction of variation.

70. Binominal distribution was introduced by ***Jacob Bernoulli,*** a Swiss mathematician.

71. Coefficient of variation is a ***relative*** measure of dispersion.

72. If correlation is zero, the two lines of regression are ***perpendicular*** to each other.

73. ***Sphere and cubes*** are generally avoided as a method of presenting data.

74. Quartile deviation is ***2/3*** of the standard deviation.

75. Replication alongwith local control reduces the ***experimental error***.

76. Multiplicative law of probability is not applicable in case of ***independent*** events.

77. Poisson distribution is the approximation of the binomial distribution if n is ***indefinitely large*** and p is ***indefinitely small.***

78. The mean of a sampling distribution of means is equal to the ***population*** mean.

79. Observations lie in the interval ì ± 2s in normal distribution curve is ***95 percent***.

80. The limit of correlation is ***-1 to +1.***

81. ANOVA was developed by ***Ronald Fisher.***

82. In normal distribution curve mean, median and mode ***coincide.***

83. In ***Poisson*** distribution mean and variance are equal.

84. If the sample size n is odd, the ***median*** is the middle terms in this array.

85. Student t-distribution was discovered by ***W.S.Gosset.***

86. In ***regression*** analysis one variable is independent and another variable is dependent on it.

87. Chi square test is also called as ***test of goodness of fit.***

88. The simplest possible measure of dispersion is ***range.***

89. ANOVA means ***analysis of variance.***

90. The most usual or predominant value in a series is called ***mode.***

91. Square root of variance is ***standard deviation.***

92. Chance of success or failure is ***probability.***

93. When there is perfect positive correlation, the value of correlation will be ***+1.***

94. Normal distribution shows ***continuous distribution.***

2

Animal Genetics and Breeding: Introduction to Computers

Q.1. True and False :

1.	True	Keyboard is an I/O device.
2.	False	Decimal number system cannot be converted into binary system.
3.	False	In the flow chart, a parallelogram is used as a connector.
4.	True	The earliest calculating device is ABACUS.
5.	True	In decimal number system base is 10 whereas in binary system the base is 2.
6.	True	ROM is a special memory in which information is permanently stored.
7.	True	Third generation computers are based on integrated circuits.
8.	False	A 3.5 inch floppy stores less data than 5.25 inch floppy.
9.	True	RAM is also known as read/write memory.
10.	True	A computer programme is a set of sequenced instructions used to direct computer to perform a required job.
11.	True	BASIC language was developed by Prof. John Kennedy and Thomas Kurtz.
12.	False	Computer virus is a living organism.
13.	False	In the first generation computer the transistors were used.

14. False Dot matrix printer is a non-impact printer.

15. True PASCAL is a high level language.

16. True UNIX is system software.

17. True MS word is application software.

18. True Various language compliers and assemblers constitute the service software.

19. True System analysts programmers and computer operators are the human ware.

20. True The discovery of zero by Indian mathematicians laid foundation stone of number system.

21. True Pascal's calculator was made by great French physicist and mathematician.

22. True The first high level language, FORTRAN was developed by IBM. (International Business Machnies Corporation)

23. False Computers are more intelligent than human being.

24. False Windows is an example of computer hardware.

25. True Group of many commands makes up a program.

26. False Rebooting means starting of a computer.

27. False A logical data is one which has a value true or false.

28. True Machine language is the only language directly understood by the computer.

29. False File on floppy disk cannot be erased and re written.

30. False The usual operating system for IBM-PC is UNIX.

31. True Floppy disk is an auxiliary memory device.

32. True Hard-disk comes under hardware.

33. True Copy is an internal DOS command.

34. False CD command is used to make the directory.

35. False Computer performs only arithmetic operations.

36. False One kilobyte is equal to 1000 bytes.

37. False In word processing package there is no use of function keys

		of key board.
38.	True	In disk operation system the DEL command is used for deleting files.
39.	False	Different types of computer have different assembly languages.
40.	True	Assembly language program requires less memory of computer in comparison to machine language.
41.	False	A magnetic tape is directly accessed.
42.	True	Peripheral devices are input output devices by which user can interact with the computer.
43.	True	Email is the cheapest and fastest mode of communication nowadays.
44.	Truc	Prcscnt day computers are based on digital technology.
45.	False	Daisy wheel printers can print graphics.
46.	True	Spread sheet packages have capabilities to create graphs and charts.
47.	True	WWW cannot incorporate multimedia.
48.	True	In the decimal number system there are ten digits from 0 to 9.
49.	True	Hardware is the mechanical and electronic device which we can see and touch.
50.	False	You can write data into ROM and read data from RAM.
51.	True	Light pen is an input device that utilizes a light sensitive detector to select objects on a display screen.
52.	True	OMR is used in tests such as aptitude tests.
53.	True	Monitor is an output unit.
54.	True	Hard disk is an auxiliary memory device.
55.	False	Operating system comes under hardware.
56.	False	FORTRAN is a low level language.
57.	False	Copy is DOS command to rename a file.
58.	False	MD command is used to change the directory.

59.	True	The printing speed of DOT matrix printers is expressed in CPS unit.
60.	False	A group of related fields is known as file.
61.	True	A flow chart is a pictorial representation of an algorithm.
62.	True	High level languages are machine independent
63.	False	A program stored in RAM is known as firmware.
64.	False	A print out copy is known as soft copy.
65.	True	Dot matrix printer does not produce solid characters.
66.	True	Ascending order of data hierarchy is byte, field, record and database.
67.	True	Assembly language is different for all types of computer.
68.	True	Word processing and database program are application softwares.
69.	False	Calculator performs both logical and arithmetic operations.
70.	False	One megabyte is equal to 1000 kilobytes.
71.	True	Very common computer language used in commercial application is COBOL.
72.	False	Hard disk of computer is the external secondary storage device.
73.	True	Computer architecture is concerned with designing and coordinating the different units in a computer
74.	False	READ statement must be followed by LET statement.
75.	False	The usual operating system for IBM-PC is UNIX.
76.	True	Microprocessor is CPU of a personal computer.
77.	False	The present day computers are based on analog technology.
78.	True	Age of a person is numeric data.
79.	True	A window environment permits a user to run several programs simultaneously and transfer data between them.
80.	False	The first computer using programme stored in its memory was electronic numerical integrator and computer.
81.	False	ALU act as a central nervous system of a computer.

82. True Optical disks are also known as write once read often disks.

83. True A flow chart shows the logical sequence in which the steps are to be performed.

84. False A dot matrix printer is used to get good quality drawings, charts and graphs.

85. False A hard disk has same storing capacity as a floppy disk.

86. True Program made available on hardware are known as firm ware.

87. False Internet is made of words inter and net, which means within networks.

88. True World Wide Web (WWW) is an information initiative, which aims to provide access to large number of documents.

89. False Computer viruses damage computer hardware.

90. True SPSS computer software is used for data analysis.

91. False Computer monitor is an input device.

92. True John von Neumann is considered as father of modern computer.

93. True Computer is made up of several components and cannot do anything itself.

Q.2. Multiple Questions :

1. The transistors were first used in:

   a. First generation computers

   b. Second generation computers

   c. Third generation computers

   d. Fourth generation computers

2. CPU consists of:

   a. ALU and storage unit

   b. ALU and output unit

   c. ALU and CPU

   d. ALU and console

3. Which of the following is a I/O device:
   a. Console b. Printer
   c. Floppy disk **d. All of the above**
4. A real variable name has:
   a. Fixed values without decimals **b. Values with decimals**
   c. Both of the above d. None of the above
5. Which of the following number system has base as 8:
   a. Binary **b. Octal**
   c. Hexadecimal d. Decimal
6. Which of the following is not a data storage device:
   a. Floppy b. Magnetic disc
   c. Winchester disc **d. Printer**
7. DOS is a:
   a. Programme **b. Operating system**
   c. Subroutine d. CPU
8. The full expression of Ics is:
   a. Integrated circuits b. International code
   c. Intelligent computers d. None of the above
9. In computer programming symbol used for multiplication is:
   a. * b. /
   c. + d. **
10. Arithmetic IF statement is used as:
   a. End statement
   b. Control statement used in decision making
   c. Declaration statement
   d. No use
11. Which of the following expression is correct:
   a. ((a+b)/c)) b. **((a+b)/c)**
   c. ((a)+(b)/c) d. All of the above

12. Which of the following expression is correct:

a. A*BC=AXB^{c}** b. (A*B)**C=A^{B}XC

c. A*B**C = (AXB) XC d. A*B**C = (AXBXCXC)

13. Which of the following is not an integer variable name:

a. INAME b. JNAME

c. KNAE **d. ANAME**

14. National informatics centre is located at:

a. Calcutta b. Mumbai

c. New Delhi d. Hyderabad

15. In FORTRAN the expression used for greater than is:

a. GT. b. >

c. < d. GT

16. In DOS the command for copying a file is:

a. </: copy filename new filename

b. >/: copy filename

c. >/: copy new filename

d. >/: copy filename filename

17. The set of pre recorded instructions executed by a computer is called the:

a. Action b. Hardware

c. Program d. Message

18. The actual machinery in a computer is called:

a. Machinery **b. Hardware**

c. Software d. Flesh ware

19. The major components of a computer are:

a. Memory b. CPU

c. I/O devices **d. All of the above**

20. A group of 8 bits is called:

a. Octave **b. Byte**

c. Nibble d. None of the above

21. The first generation of computing was in the year:
    a. 1945-1956
    b. 1956-1963
    c. 1964-1971
    d. None of the above
22. The two parts of the CPU are:
    a. Control unit and Memory
    b. Control unit and ALU
    c. Addresses and control unit
    d. Addresses and ALU
23. CPU stands for:
    a. Central Production Unit
    b. Critical Power Unit
    c. Central Processing Unit
    d. Critical Processing Unit
24. How many characters can be coded in ASCII:
    a. 7
    b. 128
    c. 256
    d. 500
25. A digital computer is better than an analog computer in terms of:
    a. Accuracy
    b. Versatility
    c. Cost
    d. All of the above
26. The central processing unit of a digital computer consists of:
    a. Arithmetic and logic unit
    b. Main memory
    c. Control unit
    d. All of the above
27. The data processing cycle consists of:
    a. Input device
    b. Central processor
    c. Output device
    d. All of the above
28. A computer system consists of:
    a. Input, out put unit
    b. Memory and control unit
    c. Arithmetic and logical unit
    d. All of the above
29. Main memory unit of a computer:
    a. Stores bulk of data and instructions
    b. Stores a small amount of data and instructions
    c. Performs arithmetic
    d. Supervises the working of all the units

30. The high level language FORTRAN is generally used for:
    a. Business
    b. General purpose applications
    c. Scientific application
    d. Process control
31. A sample is called small sample when N is:
    a. Greater than 30 **b. Less than 30**
    c. Both of the above d. None of the above
32. Critical values of Z for two tailed test at 0.05 level of significance is:
    a. -1.96 and 1.96 b. -2.81 and 2.81
    c. -2.58 and 2.58 d. None of the above
33. The program stored on ROM is called:
    a. Software b. Hardware
    c. Firmware d. None of the above
34. Which of the following is not an operating system:
    a. MS-DOS b. UNIX
    c. Windows **d. COBOL**
35. Which of the following is a part of the CPU:
    a. Printer b. Keyboard
    c. Mouse **d. Arithmetic logic unit**
36. A collection of eight bits is called:
    a. Byte b. Word
    c. Record d. File
37. A computer program consists of:
    a. System flowchart b. Program flowchart
    c. Discrete logical steps d. None of the above

38. Two kinds of main memory are:

a. ROM and RAM **b. Primary and secondary**

c. Floppy disk and hard disk d. None of the above

39. RAM is used as a short memory because:

a. **It is volatile** b. It is very expensive

c. It has small capacity d. It is programmable

40. What does ROM stand for:

a. Read only memory b. Read of memory

c. Roll of memory d. Read office manager

41. Browse command in DBASE can be used for:

a. Appending records b. Editing records

c. Both of the above d. None of the above

42. The most widely used high-level language for microcomputers is:

a. COBOL b. C

c. BASIC d. FORTRAN

43. The number of children in a family is a:

a. Analog **b. Digital**

c. Hybrid quantity d. None of the above

44. Machine language is:

a. High level language **b. Binary number**

c. ASCII system d. None of the above

45. Ascending order of data hierarchy is:

a. bit, byte, record, file database and field

b. bit, field, byte, record and file database

c. **bit, byte, field, record and file database**

d. bit, byte, record, file field and database

46. dBASE, word star, word perfect, and page maker are:

a. System software

b. Application software

c. High level programming languages

d. Low level programming languages

47. A digital computer is based on the principle of:

a. Measurement | **b. Counting**

c. Both of the above | d. None of the above

48. Which of the following is not an output device:

a. Printer | b. Monitor

c. Keyboard | d. Plotter

49. One kilobyte is equal to:

a. 1000 bits | b. 1024 bites

c. 1000 bytes | d. 1024 bytes

50. Characteristics of external storage devices are:

a. Nonvolatile | b. Reusable

c. Cheap | **d. All of the above**

51. Which of the following is not considered as a portable computer:

a. Laptop computer | b. Notebook computer

c. Palmtop computer | **d. Minicomputer**

52. The maximum different numbers a 16-bit binary signal can represent is:

a. 256 | b. 4096

c. 16384 | **d. 65536**

53. Which of the following is not an operating system:

a. UNIX | b. DOS

c. PASCAL | d. Windows

54. A computer program written in a high level language is called a:

a. Source program | b. Object program

c. Machine language program | d. None of the above

55. The radix of the binary number system is:

a. 0 | b. 8

c. 2 | d. 10

56. An input device that is used widely in supermarket is:

a. Keyboard b. Mouse

c. Track ball **d. Bar code reader**

57. Which of the following is a non impact printer:

a. Laser b. Inkjet

c. Dot matrix d. Daisy wheel

58. Which of the following is a virus vaccine:

a. Happy 2002 b. Brain

c. Dot matrix **d. Norton**

59. Which has the maximum storing capacity:

a. Floppy disk **b. Hard disk**

c. C.D. d. Zip disk

60. Who is referred as the "Father of computer":

a. Abacus **b. Charles Babbage**

c. Joseph Jacquard d. Pascal

61. Smallest unit of memory is:

a. Megabyte b. Gigabyte

c. Bit d. Kilobyte

62. A modern digital computer uses:

a. Binary system b. Octal system

c. Decimal system d. None of the above

63. MS-DOS is:

a. Operating system b. Programming language

c. Hardware d. Utility programme

64. DIR is:

a. Internal DOS command b. External DOS command

c. Command of BASIC language d. Command of FORTRAN language

65. COBOL is a :

a. **High level language** b. Machine language
c. Assembly language d. Application software

66. CD command is used :

a. For creating a new directory **b. For changing directory**
c. For erasing directory d. For copying a directory

67. Scanner is :

a. An output device **b. An input device**
c. Both a & b d. None of the above

68. Best quality print outs are obtained by:

a. Dot matrix printer b. Inkjet printer
c. Laser printer d. Line printer

69. The latest versions of PC are:

a. PCAT-286 b. PCAT-386
c. PCAT-486 **d. Pentium**

70. A file extension cannot have more than:

a. **3 characters** b. 8 characters
c. 4 characters d. 6 characters

71. A digital computer is based on the principle of:

a. Measurement **b. Counting**
c. Both of the above d. None of the above

72. Which of the following is not an input device:

a. Scanner **b. Monitor**
c. Keyboard d. Mouse

73. Primary memory in comparison to secondary storage is:

a. Costly b. Limited capacity
c. Faster **d. All of the above**

74. MS Word is a :

a. Operating system software **b. Application software**

c. Assembler d. None of the above

75. Relational operators are :

a. Addition and multiplication b. AND, OR and NOT

c. >, < and = d. None of the above

76. Majority of the computers in the world are of :

a. Analog type **b. Digital type**

c. Hybrid type d. None of the above

77. Which of the following is an impact printer:

a. Laser b. Inkjet

c. Dot matrix d. Plotter

78. Which of the following is an example of volatile memory:

a. ROM **b. RAM**

c. EPROM d. PROM

79. Larger unit of memory is expressed in:

a. Kilobyte b. Gigabyte

c. Megabyte **d. All of the above**

80. In limnaea, the dextral type shell coiling is:

a. Right **b. Left**

c. Dorsal left d. Ventral left

81. Compound may be:

a. Digital **b. Analog**

c. Hybrid d. All of the above

82. A system that links a number of stand alone computers together is:

a. A network b. Multiprocessing

c. A pipeline d. None of the above

83. What does RAM stand for :

a. Read any memorandum
b. Random access memory
c. Random allot memory
d. None of the above

84. Which one of the following computer programming language:

a. BASIC
b. CRD
c. ALU
d. CPU

85. Algorithm means:

a. Taking logarithm of some variable
b. Processing data by computer in a rhythmic fashion
c. Solving problem with logically defined procedure
d. Solving problem with the help of a computer

86. Storage medium used in second generation of computers was:

a. Magnetic drum
b. Magnetic core
c. Magnetic disk
d. All of the above

87. Processing of data includes:

a. Storing
b. Computing
c. Retrieving
d. All of the above

88. Introduction of computers can be considered in IT:

a. First revolution
b. Second revolution
c. Third revolution
d. Fourth revolution

89. CAM needs:

a. Computer
b. Robotics
c. Both of the above
d. None of the above

90. CAD is used for:

a. Creating designs
b. Modifying designs
c. Selecting designs
d. All of the above

91. Which one of the following is not an operating system:

a. DOS
b. UNIX
c. WINDOWS
d. COBOL

92. The most common output device is:

a. Plotter b. Printer

c. Fax machine **d. Monitor**

93. The first electronic computer was:

a. UNIVAC-I **b. ENIAC**

c. MARK-I d. IBM-70

94. Diagram and graphs are the tools of:

a. Collection of data b. Analysis of data

c. Presentation of data d. None of the above

95. Main memory transfer information to:

a. ALU b. Output unit

c. Control unit d. Main memory unit

96. Computer system consists of:

a. Input output unit b. Memory unit

c. Arithmetic and logic unit **d. All of the above**

97. A floppy disk is:

a. A second generation invention

b. Expensive than the magnetic tape

c. Used with large computers

d. None of the above

98. Which of the following is a secondary storage device:

a. Magnetic disk b. Plotter

c. MICR d. OMR

99. Speech input system can convert :

a. As many words as possible in to human language

b. A limited number of words in to human language

c. Human voice to machine language

d. None of the above

100. Multiple choice examination answer sheets are evaluated by :

a. Magnetic tape radar

b. Magnetic ink character reader

c. Optical mark reader

d. Optical character reader

101. Which of the following is not a storage device :

a. Floppy
b. Compact disk
c. Punched card
d. Light pen

102. The brain of the computer is:

a. ROM
b. ALU
c. CPU
d. RAM

103. Which of the following is not an input device:

a. Key board
b. Mouse
c. Printer
d. Joy stick

104. Which of the following is not a web browser:

a. Adobe page maker
b. Netscape communicator
c. Internet explorer
d. Netscape navigator

105. In internet terminology.com means:

a. Commerce
b. Cyber
c. Commercial organization
d. Computer

106. URL stands for:

a. Uniform research loader

b. Uniform resource locator

c. Uniform resource loader

d. None of the above

107. Which one of the following computer languages has of highest level:

a. BASIC
b. PASCAL
c. C++
d. All of the above

108. Binary number system used only two digits:

a. 0 and 1 | b. 0 and 2
c. 1 and 1 | d. 1 and 2

109. When you open internet, the first page is referred to as:

a. Master page | **b. Home page**
c. First page | d. All of the above

110. A data base is a:

a. Collection of related files | b. Collection of related fields
c. Collection of related records | **d. All of the above**

111. Storage device of computer includes:

a. Microprocessor | b. Integrated circuit
c. Transistors | **d. Hard disk**

112. Measure of dispersion includes:

a. Standard deviation | b. Mean deviation
c. Range | **d. All of the above**

113. Monitor is:

a. Operating system | **b. Hardware**
c. Software | d. Input device

114. An electronic digital computer is a machine used for:

a. Storage of data and instructions
b. For mathematical calculations and data processing
c. For performing repetitive calculations
d. All of the above

Q3. Fill in the blanks :

1. The full expression of PCAT ***personal computer advance technology***.
2. The full expression of DBMS is ***data base management system.***
3. Full expression of e-mail is ***electronic mail***.
4. In computers the data is stored in the form of ***file*** having specific names.

5. The relational operators are ***GT, GE, LT, LE, EQ and NE***.
6. In flow chart a circle symbolizes as **connector.**
7. ALU stands for ***Arithmetic logic unit*.**
8. ASCII stands ***American standard code for information interchange.***
9. Integer variable names start with ***IJKLMN.***
10. Computer machinery parts and accessories are called as ***hardware*.**
11. The particular code used by user to prevent the access to his directories/ file by other users is called as ***password*.**
12. In flow chart a rectangle is used for ***process***.
13. Full expression of MS-DOS is ***Microsoft Disk Operating System.***
14. The logical operators are ***AND., OR., NOT***.
15. In third generation computers the transistors are replaced by ***silicon chip.***
16. ENIAC stands for ***electronic numeric integrator and calculator*** was developed first electronic computer.
17. The important applications of computers are ***business, scientific, engineering, metrological, graphic and space research*.**
18. Four important advantages of computers are ***speed, volume, accuracy and complexity.***
19. Longest key in the last row of the key board is ***space bar.***
20. Four key parts that supports a computer are ***input unit, memory, processor, output unit.***
21. ***Magnetic disk*** device can act as an input and output device.
22. The key used to enter a command is called ***enter key.***
23. The body cells of the individual are ***diploid*.**
24. ***CPU*** is called heart and nerve center of a digital computer.
25. ALU looks after the mathematical and ***logical*** operation.
26. A set of similar record is called a ***file*.**
27. In general a byte consists of ***8*** bits.
28. The component of a computer which stores information is called ***primary memory.***

29. Information from auxiliary memory is transferred to ALU via ***main memory or primary memory.***
30. The word FORTRAN stand for ***formula translation.***
31. The word BASIC means ***Beginner's All Purpose Symbolic Instruction Code.***
32. ***Skewness*** is the degree of asymmetry of a distribution.
33. **ABACUS** is the first known calculating device.
34. The binary system has ***two*** digits.
35. User can communicate with computer through ***input*** devices.
36. The translation of source program into machine language is called as ***compiler.***
37. The longest key used to put blank in a line is called as ***space bar.***
38. Computers are mostly used in office for ***word processing.***
39. The processing speed of a computer is measured in ***MHz.***
40. ***Serial*** port is used to connect the system with mouse.
41. Scanner is an ***input*** unit.
42. The software that converts the assembly language into machine language is called ***assembler.***
43. 1MB is equal to ***1024*** kilo-bytes.
44. ***Del*** is the DOS command which can delete a file.
45. ***Space bar*** key is used to create space.
46. **ROM** is a permanent memory in computer.
47. ***Assembler*** is a computer program which converts the assembly language instructions in to object code.
48. Personal computer is also referred to as ***microcomputer.***
49. A collection of 8 bits is called ***bytes.***
50. The DEL command in MS-DOS is used for deleting ***files.***
51. Machine language is ***low*** level language.
52. The process of detecting and correcting errors in computer programme is known as ***debugging.***

53. Putting instructions and data into the computer system is known as ***input.***
54. In flowchart, ***parallelogram*** is used to represent input and output operations.
55. The only two characters used in machine language are ***0 and 1.***
56. ***Window*** is a graphical user interface (GUI) based operating system.
57. Vacuum tubes were used in ***first*** generation computers.
58. Arithmetic logic unit (ALU) is a part of ***CPU.***
59. Two main classes of the software are ***system soft ware*** and ***application software.***
60. The four categories of digital computers are ***mini computer, micro computer, mainframes and super computer.***
61. DRAM stands for ***dynamic read access memory.***
62. A device that controls the movements of the cursor or pointer on a display screen is called the ***mouse.***
63. COBOL stands for ***common business oriented language.***
64. ***E-mail*** is an electronic message send from one computer to another.
65. OLE stands for ***object Linking & Embedding.***
66. Binary number system uses only two digits ***0*** and ***1.***
67. A computer consists of input unit, output unit and ***CPU.***
68. ***Floppy disc*** is an input as well output unit.
69. The software that converts the high level language into machine language step by step is called ***Interpretator.***
70. 1KB is equal to ***1000*** bytes.
71. ***CLS*** is the DOS command which can clear the screen.
72. ***Space bar*** is the longest key of keyboard.
73. **RAM** is a temporary memory in computer.
74. Coefficient of coincidence=% of observed double crossover divided by ***% expected double crossover.***
75. In flowchart, ***diamond*** rhombus box is used to denote decision.
76. VLSI stands for ***very large scale interaction.***

77. ***Charles Babbage*** is known as father of computer.
78. Variances are expressed in ***squared*** units.
79. The correlation coefficient between two independent variables is ***zero.***
80. Two events are ***independent*** if occurrence of one does not affect probability of occurrence of other.
81. All experimental units in a block must be treated as ***similarly/uniformly*** as possible.
82. Bioassays are used to determine the potency of a test preparation to that of ***standard*** preparation.
83. ***Debugging*** is process of detecting and correcting errors in the computer softwares.
84. The oval shaped symbol in a flow chart is an indication of ***starter end.***
85. ***Compilers*** translate the source program into an executable program.
86. Machine language programs require ***low*** memory of computer in comparison to assembly language.
87. Microcomputer belongs to ***third*** generation of computer.
88. Input/Output symbol in flowchart is represented by ***parallelogram*****.**
89. ***Cursor*** is a mark that shows you are on the display unit.
90. One gigabyte is= ***10^8*** bytes.
91. Transistor was used as ***second*** generation computers.
92. FORTRAN stands for ***formula translator*****.**
93. The two types of plotters are ***Flat belt*** type and ***drum type.***
94. ***Control unit and ALU*** of the computer system is jointly known as CPU.
95. Flow chart consists of boxes called ***symbol*** and arrows called ***flow lines.***
96. A punch card consists of ***80*** *r*ows columns.
97. The smallest unit of data in a binary system is ***bit.***
98. A part of the central processing unit that does mathematical calculations and makes logical decision is ***arithmetic logic unit.***
99. BASIC stands for ***Beginners All Purpose Symbolic Instruction Code.***
100. HTTP stands for ***hyper text transfer protocol*****.**

101. RAM sands for ***random access memory*.**
102. The database saved in MS Access takes ***mdb*** extension.
103. DBMS stands for ***Database Management System*.**
104. The keyboard, VDU and printer are all connected to the ***CPU.***
105. Data is fed into the computer through ***keyboard.***
106. LAN stands for ***local area network.***
107. The ***computer*** performs mathematical calculations and logical operations.
108. CPU means ***central processing unit.***
109. FORTRAN is an example of ***high*** level language.
110. IBM-PC is a ***micro*** computer.

3

Animal Genetics and Breeding Livestock Breeding System

Q.1. True & False:

1. <u>True</u> Mule is the cross of male Ass *Equinus asinus* with female horse *(Equinus caballus)*.
2. <u>False</u> Inbreeding cannot be used for the development of distinct lines or families.
3. <u>True</u> Recessive genes appear in homozygous form with inbreeding.
4. <u>False</u> Continuous use of purebred sire on nondescript female is called out crossing.
5. <u>True</u> In cross breeding maximum hetrozygosity is possible in first generation.
6. <u>True</u> Common ancestor is the individual common in pedigree of two individuals.
7. <u>True</u> In case of full brother-sister mating, increase in homozygosity is less than half as compared to self fertilization in plants.
8. <u>False</u> In grading up, local population becomes almost purebred after four generation.
9. <u>True</u> Significant difference in egg production among populations reared under identical conditions of management and feeding is an indication of genetic differences among them.
10. <u>True</u> The main advantage of 3-way or 4-way cross is to overcome the reproductive disadvantage.

11.	False	Mating of the two inbred lines belonging to different breeds is called incrossing.
12.	False	Inbreeding increases the number of recessive alleles in the population.
13.	False	Traits governed by dominance, over dominance or epistatic gene action will not be affected adversely by inbreeding.
14.	False	Heterosis is much more evident in characters of high heritability.
15.	False	While evolving inbred lines inbreeding should be intense in the beginning.
16.	True	The theory of path coefficient was given by Wright.
17.	True	Inbred animals are usually less able to cope with the environment than noninbred animals.
18.	True	Heterosis occurs generally when unrelated genotypes are crossed.
19.	False	Heterosis is higher in backcrosses than the three way and four way crosses.
20.	False	Strain crosses within a breed generally exhibit more heterosis than breed crosses.
21.	True	The half-sib mating would be the closest possible mating in a line breeding programme.
22.	True	Formation of lines will be most useful for less hereditary characters.
23.	True	Normally amount of heterosis shown in F_2 is only half as great as shown in F_1.
24.	True	Inbreeding affects all independent pairs of segregating genes in the same way.
25.	False	Inbreeding cannot be used alongwith selection to uncover and estimate recessive genes.
26.	True	Heterosis shown by F_2 is only half as that shown by F_1.
27.	False	Two way flow of genes is possible in closed nucleus breeding system.

28. True Out crossing is the mating of unrelated animal within the same pure breed.
29. False Grading up produces purebred in 5 to 6 generations.
30. True Reproductive efficiency decreases in inbred animal.
31. True Heterosis will be more if number of breeds involved in cross breeding are more.
32. True Inbreeding does not increase the number of recessive alleles in a population.
33. True The traits associated with physical fitness are improved by crossbreeding.
34. False Holstein Friesian breed of cattle is preferred for crossbreeding in hilly areas.
35. False The crossbreeding results in sheep for improving wool quality are very encouraging.
36. True Avikalin and Avivastra were produced by crossbreeding.
37. True Hinny is result of species hybridization.
38. True Random mating is a haphazard type of breeding.
39. False In top crossing individuals from two breeds are mated.
40. True Most efficient form of inbreeding is selfing.
41. True Inbreeding is used for fixation of genes.
42. False Inbreeding changes the gene frequency of desirable genes only.
43. False Heritability may also be obtained by calculating repeatability of the trait.
44. False Close breeding produced progenies are more variable than outbreeding.
45. False Heritability is the same in all herds for a given trait.
46. False The coefficient of relationship between parent and offspring is always one.
47. True Genetic effect of out crossing and crossbreeding is same.
48. False Outbreed individuals breed true.

49.	False	Cattlo is the cross of bison and zebra.
50.	True	Increase in homozygosity due to inbreeding is irrespective of kind of gene action.
51.	False	Out breeding effects are more for traits affected by additive genes.
52.	False	Outbreed parents are more likely to be proponent.
53.	False	The admired ancestor in line breeding is always a female.
54.	False	Mating of inbred females with unrelated male is topcrossing.
55.	True	Epistasis is the interaction between pairs of genes that are not alleles.
56.	True	Outbreeding is used to introduce desirable genes in the population lacking them.
57.	True	Regular crossing exploit both additive and non-additive gene effects.
58.	True	Traits governed by over dominance show decrease in mean under inbreeding.
59.	True	Though the phenotypic value of a trait is increased by crossbreeding, the breeding value is reduced.
60.	False	The absence of heterosis is the sufficient ground for concluding that the individual loci show no dominance.
61.	True	Inbred hybrids are the progeny produced from one inbred line and one non-inbred line.
62.	True	The genetic effects of line breeding are the same as those of inbreeding.
63.	False	Prepotency will decrease as the inbreeding increases.
64.	True	Inbred individuals often show more environmental variation than non-inbred individuals.
65.	False	Cross breeding creates individuals which breed true.
66.	True	The greater the genetic difference in the parent the hybrid vigor in the offspring will be greater.
67.	False	There is more gain by using four breeds cross over a three breed cross.

68. False Through embryo transfer technology we can use more efficiently the breeding bull.

69. True Hybrid vigor applies to the progeny from the crossing of strains, breeds, varieties or species.

70. False Crossbreeding is useful when the traits are governed by additive gene action.

71. True Inbreeding depression depends on the rate of inbreeding, gene frequency and level of dominance.

72. False Inbreeding should be practiced in commercial herd.

73. True The outward effect of inbreeding will depend upon the genes present in the stock with which breeding began.

74. True Commercial herds are not allowed for inbreeding.

75. False Milk production is a qualitative trait.

76. False Rotational crossing is more common in cattle.

77. True Crossbred are more suspectable to disease in comparison to indigenous breed.

78. False In case of crossbreeding same two breeds are required.

79. True Inbreeding coefficient is a measure of homozygosity.

80. True The *"Pian niu"* is produced by crossing cattle and yak.

81. True Outbreeding increases heterozygosity.

82. True High heritability shows high correlation between genotype and phenotype.

83. False Mating between two different breeds is termed species hybridization.

84. True The amount of heterosis is expressed as the difference between the F_1 and the mid parent value.

85. True Crossbreeding evolves new breeds.

86. False Good inbred animals never show prepotency.

87. False The degree of relationship between parent and offspring is 25 percent.

88. False Inbreeding makes only desirable genes homozygous.

89.	True	Half sibs have collateral relationship.
90.	True	Generally heterozygotes are better protected.
91.	False	Line breeding produces offspring more variable than out breeding.
92.	False	Principles of inheritance for qualitative and quantitative traits are different.
93.	False	Individuals having same inbreeding coefficient are homozygous for same loci.
94.	True	The inbreeding leads to expression of recessive genes.
95.	True	Holstein crosses are superior for milk than Jersey crosses.
96.	False	Brown swiss crosses are superior for reproductive efficiency than Jersey crosses.
97.	False	Milk production show high heterosis.
98.	False	The coefficient of relationship between identical twins is 0.50.
99.	False	Crossbred sire is more prepotent than pure-bred.
100.	False	Artificial insemination is popular in pigs.
101.	True	Artificial insemination increases selection differential.
102.	False	Mating between half bred and half bred is called close breeding.
103.	True	Service period is period between parturition and conception.
104.	True	Mongrel is a result of accidental mating.
105.	False	Crossbreeding is mating between unrelated animals of same breed.
106.	True	*Pien niu* is product of *Bos indicus* male and *Bos grunniens*.
107.	True	Calving interval is the interval between two successive calving.
108.	True	Heterosis is decreased by half in F2 generation.
109.	False	Relationship coefficient for half sib is 50 percent.
110.	True	In criss crossing two breeds are mated alternatively.
111.	True	Hybridization is the extreme form of outbreeding.
112.	True	Relationship coefficient for mating of full sister and full brother is 0.25.

113. True — Inbreeding do not cause any drastic change for commercial purpose.

114. False — Top crossing is cross of non-descript breed with a recognized breed.

115. True — Low heritability indicates the poor breeding value.

116. True — Test cross is mating between F_1 with one of its parents.

117. False — Heterosis occurs due to intensive inbreeding.

118. True — Species hybridization is an example of widest possible outbreeding.

119. False — Variances due to dominance and epistatic deviations are easy to estimate.

120. False — Maximum hetrozygosity is possible in second and third generation.

121. False — Positive assartative mating increases hetrozygosity.

122. False — The fluctuations of gene frequency with inbreeding in large population would be less extreme as compare to small populations.

123. False — Inbreeding coefficient of an individual is equal to the relationship between the parents of the individual.

124. False — The proportion of heterozygotes pairs of genes decreases with outbreeding.

125. True — The coefficient of relationship between an individual and its double first cousins is 0.125 percent.

126. True — Diallel is a system of mating among all possible combinations.

127. True — Full exploitation of maternal, paternal and individual heterosis is possible in four ways cross.

128. False — Inbreeding depression is maximum in trait governed by additive genes.

129. False — Assortative mating and inbreeding are same.

130. True — Inbreeding is usually used for production of seed stock.

131. False — Coefficient or relationship between double first cousins is 6.25 percent.

132. True — Line breeding is used to concentrate the inheritance of an outstanding ancestor among its descendants.

133. False — Advantages of heterosis cannot be obtained from crossbreeding.

134. True — Quantitative characters are strongly modified by environmental variation.

135. True — Concept of effective population size is useful for comparing populations with different structures.

136. True — Best linear unbiased prediction (BLUP) is a method of predicting expected breeding value of the individual.

137. True — The inbreeding coefficient of an individual is half the relationship between its parents.

138. False — Inbreeding changes both gene and genotype frequencies of the population.

139. False — Inbred lines are less likely to breed true than the out breeds.

140. True — Small and closed herd is always inbred herd after few generations.

141. False — Criss crossing is the use of sires of three breeds in rotation on crossbred females.

142. False — Inbreeding cannot be used for the development of *Equis caballus*.

143. True — Full brother-sister mating is the most intense from of inbreeding in animals.

144. False — Parent offspring mating are not equal to full brother sister mating.

145. False — The term heterosis was coined by William Batson.

146. False — Coefficient of inbreeding ranges from -1 to+1.

147. True — In crossbreeding maximum productivity depends upon full advantage of heterosis and the frequency of desirable genes with additive effects.

148. True — Fluctuation of the gene frequency with inbreeding in large population would be less extreme as compared to small population.

149. False — Epistasis can be fixed in a single line or breed.

Q.2. Multiple Choices Questions

1. The mating system which increases heterozygosity is called:

   a. Inbreeding b. Line breeding

   c. Outbreeding d. None of the above

2. Ability of an individual to stamp its own characteristics in the offspring is called:

   a. Prepotency b. Heterosis

   c. Overdominance d. None of the above

3. The indigenous breeds of cattle used at various centers of AICRP on cattle are:

   a. Hariana and Ongole **b. Hariana, Gir and Ongole**

   c. Gir and Ongole d. None of the above

4. The exotic breeds of cattle used at various centers of AICRP on cattle are:

   a. Jersey and Brown Swiss

   b. Brown Swiss and Holstein Friesian

   c. Jersey, Brown Swiss and Holstein Friesian

   d. None of the above

5. Central Institute of Buffalo Research is located at :

   a. Karnal b. Bangalore

   c. Hisar d. IVRI, Izatnagar

6. In embryo transfer technology follicle stimulating hormone (FSH) is used for:

   a. Short term storage of embryo b. Long term storage of embryo

   c. Super ovulation d. None of the above

7. When any individual of one sex has an equal chance of mating with any other individual the mating system is known as:

   a. Random mating b. Outbreeding

   c. Inbreeding d. None of the above

8. When all available lines are crossed in all possible combinations the system is known as:

   a. Recurrent selection **b. Diallel crossing**

   c. Both of the above d. None of the above

9. Heterosis is caused due to:

   a. Dominance b. Over dominance

   c. Epistasis **d. All of the above**

10. System of mating in which higher relationship is maintained with a favoured ancestor in subsequent generations:

    a. Close inbreeding b. Out breeding

    c. Line breeding d. None of the above

11. A female ass is also known as:

    a. Jack **b. Jennet**

    c. Mule d. None of the above

12. The variance–covariance method for the estimation of inbreeding coefficient was given by:

    a. Wright **b. Malecot**

    c. Fisher d. None of the above

13. Majority of breeds of cattle in India are:

    a. Dairy breed **b. Draught breed**

    c. Dual breed d. All of the above

14. Selection limit means a stage when there is no:

    a. Genetic variation b. Phenotypic variation

    c. Further response to selection d. Selection differential

15. If achieving homozygosity in a population is the desired goal, how you will breed the individuals:

    a. Random mating b. Assortative mating

    c. Breeding the close relatives d. None of the above

16. Mating of two unrelated animals of the same breed is called:

a. Grading up
b. Inbreeding
c. Outcrossing
d. Line breeding

17. Breeding system which is designed to take advantage of good qualities of two breeds:

a. Cross breeding
b. Grading up
c. Heterosis
d. Line breeding

18. When the performance of the cross not only exceeds the mid parent but also the better parent, the performance is known as:

a. Dominance
b. Over dominance
c. Both of the above
d. None of the above

19. The development strategy followed in breeding tract of pure buffaloes is:

a. Grading up
b. Selective breeding
c. Cross breeding
d. Inbreeding

20. Who is the father of modern scientifi Animal Breeding:

a. T.H.Morgan
b. L.M.Winter
c. J.L.Lush
d. C.R.Handerson

21. Mating of distantly related animals with an aim of maintaining relationship to an outstanding sire is:

a. Inbreeding
b. Line breeding
c. Close breeding
d. Grading up

22. Percentage of relationship between identical twin is:

a. 0.5
b. One
c. More than one
d. Zero

23. Systematic cross breeding using three or more breeds is called:

a. Criss crossing
b. Rotational crossing
c. Grading up
d. Species hybridization

24. For the production of heterosis the most important genes involved are:

a. Additive genes
b. Dominant genes
c. Non-additive genes
d. Sex linked genes

25. Criss crossing is a form of:

a. Cross breeding **b. Back crossing**

c. Top crossing d. Out crossing

26. An inbreeding coefficient of 50% will be attained by half sib mating after:

a. One generation b. Two generation

c. Three generation **d. More than five generation**

27. The progeny of a single individual obtained by selfing is known as:

a. Full sib b. Clone

c. Half sib **d. Pure line**

28. Inbreeding depression is a consequence due to change in:

a. Genotype frequency b. Gene frequency

c. Genetic variability d. Phenotypic variability

29. The coefficient of relationship is most accurately defined as a measure of:

a. Proportion of genes, which are homozygous in two individuals.

b. Probable likeness of the genotype of two individuals

c. Proportion of genes that two individuals have in common by descent

d. None of the above

30. On theoretical grounds it appears to be impossible to obtain a highly vigrous homozygotes as heterozygotes, if vigor was due to:

a. Dominance b. Additive gene action

c. Over dominance d. Interaction of non-allelic loci

31. Under self fertilization the proportion of heterozygotes in a population is reduced each generation by:

a. 1/2 b. 1/4

c. 1/6 d. 1/7

32. The cross breeding combines desirable traits of:

a. Same breed b. Different breeds

c. Different strains d. None of the above

33. The crossing of nondescript breed with well established breed is known as:

a. Crossbreeding b. Top breeding

c. Line breeding **d. Grading up**

34. Hybrid sterility may be due to:

a. Chromosomal incompatibility b. Gene incompatibility

c. Nutritional incompatibility d. All of the above

35. Coefficient of relationship between double first cousin is:

a. 0.015 **b. 0.25**

c. 1.00 d. None of the above

36. The percentage of homozygosity in progenies produced from mating of half sibs is:

a. 25% **b. 2.5%**

c. 50% d. None of the above

37. The term coefficient of inbreeding was proposed by:

a. Falconer **b. Sewall Wright**

c. Malecot d. None of the above

38. Inbreeding leads to decline in:

a. Fertility b. Viability

c. Both of the above d. None of the above

39. When heterozygotes (Aa) is superior to either of the two homozygotes (AA or aa) the condition is called:

a. Dominance **b. Over dominance**

c. Epistasis d. None of the above

40. When crossbred females are mated to males of one of the parental breeds, the mating system take advantage of:

a. Paternal heterosis **b. Maternal heterosis**

c. Individual heterosis d. None of the above

41. When two genes arise from the direct replication of the same gene from a common ancestor, two such genes are known as:

a. Identical by descent b. Alike in state

c. Both of the above d. None of the above

42. Cross between domestic cattle and American buffalo (*Bos taurus* x *Bos bison*) is called:

a. Bantung | b. Yak
c. Cattalo | d. None of the above

43. The relationship between an offspring and one of its great grand parents is:

a. 1/4 | b. 1/16
c. ^/8 | d. ½

44. A system of breeding purebred sires of a given breed to non-descript female is called:

a. Crossbreeding | b. Crisscrossing
c. Grading-up | d. Line breeding

45. Individuals which are having common sire and dam in a pedigree are called:

a. Half sibs | **b. Full sibs**
c. Collateral relatives | d. None of the above

46. When a highly inbred tester line is crossed with large number of individual's source population, the system is called:

a. Reciprocal recurrent selection | **b. Recurrent selection**
c. Both of the above | d. None of the above

47. Higher genetic diversity between two population will give:

a. Less amount of heterosis | b. Zero heterosis
c. Higher amount of heterosis | d. None of the above

48. Frieswal strain of cattle has been developed at:

a. NDRI Karnal | b. IVRI Izatnagar
c. PDC Meerut | d. None of the above

49. The system of mating which uses sires of two breeds in rotation on crossbred females is called:

a. Rotational crossing | b. Grading
c. Synthetic | **d. Criss crossing**

50. The system of mating practiced to maintain the inheritance level in crossbred population at a constant level is:

a. Crossbreeding b. Top crossing

c. Grading **d. Intersemating**

51. Mating between two established breeds is called:

a. Rotational crossing b. Grading up

c. Crossbreeding d. Species hybridization

52. The coefficient of inbreeding after three generation of full sib mating will be:

a. 0.250 b. 0.375

c. 0.500 d. 0.594

53. Higher genetic diversity between two populations will give:

a. Less amount of heterosis b. Zero heterosis

c. Higher amount of heterosis d. None of the above

54. In a population when an individual of one sex has an equal change of mating with any other individual of the opposite sex, the system of mating is termed as:

a. Outbreeding **b. Random mating**

c. Inbreeding d. Top crossing

55. Mating of females of the non-inbred population to inbred males is known as:

a. Line breeding **b. Top crossing**

c. Forward crossing d. Inbred crossing

56. The crossbreeding is practiced to take advantage of:

a. Dominance **b. Heterosis**

c. Epistasis d. All of the above

57. Line and strain are produced by:

a. Crossbreeding b. Out crossing

c. Inbreeding d. None of the above

58. The coefficient of relationship is 100 percent between:

a. Parent of offspring
b. Brother and sister
c. Dizygotic twins
d. Monozygotic twins

59. Crossing of non-descript breed with well established breed is known as:

a. Crossbreeding
b. Top breeding
c. Line crossing
d. Grading up

60. Which of the breeding system utilizes sires from two breeds alternatively:

a. Outcrossing
b. Criss crossing
c. Rotational crossing
d. Top crossing

61. In crossing inbred lines where each line is crossed with every other line is called:

a. Top crossing
b. Diallel crossing
c. RRS
d. None of the above

62. The crossing of inbred male line with inbred female line of the same breed is known as:

a. Inbreeding
b. In crossing
c. Incrossing
d. Crossbreeding

63. Strain crossing is milder form of:

a. Crossbreeding
b. Inbreeding
c. Outbreeding
d. Line breeding

64. Inbreeding depression depends on:

a. Rate of migration
b. Rate of mutation
c. Intensity of selection
d. Level of dominance

65. Number of ancestors of an individual at n^{th} back generation will be:

a. 3^n
b. 2^n
c. 4^n
d. None of the above

66. Proportion of heterozygotes after 'n' generation of inbreeding will be:

a. 16
b. 2
c. 4
d. 0

67. Inbreeding coefficient in two generations of full sib mating will be:

a. 0.375 b. 0.275
c. 0.500 d. 0.250

68. Magnitude of inbreeding depression depends upon:

a. Gene frequency b. Inbreeding coefficient
c. Degree of dominance **d. All of the above**

69. Most mild form of inbreeding is:

a. Half sib mating b. Son-dam mating
c. Self fertilization d. Full sib mating

70. Cross of cattle and yak is called as:

a. Pian niu b. Cattalo
c. Hinny d. None of the above

71. Relationship between half sisters is:

a. 0.015 b. 1.00
c. 0.125 **d. 0.25**

72. The term inbreeding coefficient was introduced by:

a. Malecot b. Falconer
c. Hardy-Weinberg **d. None of the above**

73. Mating based on phenotypes of individual is:

a. Outbreeding b. Inbreeding
c. Assortative mating d. None of the above

74. Inbreeding increases:

a. Genetic uniformity b. Phenotypic uniformity
c. Production **d. None of the above**

75. Character insensitive to inbreeding:

a. Fitness traits b. Reproductive traits
c. Maternal traits **d. Skeletal traits**

76. The most rapid method of attaining high level of inbreeding in animal:

a. Selfing
b. Full sib mating
c. Half sib mating
d. Repeat back crossing

77. Experiments indicate that traits having bearing on fitness are depressed most by:

a. Line breeding
b. Out breeding
c. Inbreeding
d. Grading up

78. Percentage of relationship between full sib is:

a. 0.25
b. 0.50
c. 0.63
d. 0.75

79. Inbreeding uncovers:

a. Recessive genes
b. Dominant genes
c. All of the above
d. None of the above

80. The mating system in which breeding of purebred sire of a given breed is crossed with native females and their female offspring generation after generation is known as:

a. Criss-crossing
b. Rotational crossing
c. Line crossing
d. Grading up

81. A double cross is also known as:

a. One way cross
b. Two way cross
c. Three way cross
d. Four way cross

82. Cross breeding promotes the pairing of unlike genes and it is used for:

a. For the formation of new breed
b. To produce market animals
c. All of the above
d. None of the above

83. Cousin mating comes under:

a. Line breeding
b. Close breeding
c. Random mating
d. None of the above

84. One of the genetic effects of inbreeding is:

a. To change the gene frequency

b. To increase homozygosity within-line

c. To increase homozygosity between lines

d. To decrease homozygosity in all the lines

85. Mating of unrelated animals within the breed is called:

a. Out breeding **b. Out crossing**

c. Inbreeding d. Grading up

86. In the absence of epistatic inter-action heterosis observed in F_2 generation is equivalent to:

a. Same as observed in F_1

b. Twice the heterosis observed in F_1

c. Half of the heterosis observed in F_1

d. None of the above

87. The value for coefficient of inbreeding may range from:

a. 0.0 to 1.0 b. -1 to +1

c. -1 to 0 d. Any range is possible

88. An inbreeding coefficient of 50% can be achieved by:

a. Two generations of selfing

b. Three generations of full sib mating

c. Five generations of half sib mating

d. All of the above

89. Which one of the following is not affected by inbreeding depression:

a. Population mean **b. Gene frequency**

c. Genotype frequency d. Homozygosity

90. Breeding system through which the non-descript cattle can be converted to a known breed is called:

a. Crossbreeding **b. Grading up**

c. Line breeding d. Inbreeding

91. Traits sensitive to inbreeding depression have following characteristics:
    a. Low heritability b. Show large heterotic effect
    c. Related to fitness **d. All of the above**

92. Extreme form of out breeding is called:
    a. Out crossing b. Crossbreeding
    c. Species hybridization d. Grading up

93. Crossbreeding is practiced to take advantage of:
    a. Dominance **b. Heterosis**
    c. Epitasis d. Prepotency

94. Genetic basis of heterosis is:
    a. Maternal effects b. Additive gene effects
    c. Pleiotropism **d. Overdominance**

95. Rotational crossbreeding is generally practiced in:
    a. Cattle **b. Pig**
    c. Yak d. Horse

96. The most practical use of inbreeding is to:
    a. Detect sex-linked traits b. Detect heterosis
    c. Develop inbred lines d. Increase heterozygosity

97. In crossbreeding, the breeds used should be genetically:
    a. Close b. Very close
    c. Distant d. All of the above

98. Random mating is done to:
    a. Increase the prepotency
    b. Change the genetic constitution of population
    c. Keep the genetic constitution of the population unchanged
    d. Increased heterosis

99. Decline in the performance will be more as a result of inbreeding when traits are effected greatly by:
    a. Additive gene action **b. Non-additive gene action**
    c. Multiple allele d. All of the above

100. The offspring produced by crossing of a stallion and a female donkey is know as:

a.	Mule	b.	Cattalo
c.	**Hinny**	d.	Jennet

101. Like to like mating system is called as:

a.	**Assortative mating**	b.	Criss crossing
c.	Rotational crossing	d.	Top crossing

102. The new breeds can be evolved by:

a.	Inbreeding	b.	Line breeding
c.	Out crossing	**d.**	**Crossbreeding**

103. Under AICRP on cattle, which of the following exotic breed was not considered in evolving new dairy cattle breed:

a.	Holstein Friesian	b.	Jersey
c.	Brown Swiss	**d.**	**Ayrshire**

104. Extreme form of cross breeding is:

a.	Criss crossing	**b.**	**Hybridization**
c.	Rotational crossing	d.	Top crossing

105. Strain crossing is the milder form of:

a.	Inbreeding	**b.**	**Cross breeding**
c.	Top crossing	d.	Line breeding

106. Inbreeding depression would be maximum for the traits related to:

a.	Fat content	**b.**	**Reproduction**
c.	Growth	d.	Carcass

107. Heterozygote superiority is due to:

a.	Pleiotropism	b.	Multiple gene action
c.	**Over dominance**	d.	Additive gene action

108. Which of the breeding system utilizes sires from more than two breeds:

a.	Out crossing	b.	Criss crossing
c.	**Rotational crossing**	d.	Top crossing

109. In flock of poultry, 50 cockerels are mated with 200 pullets, the rate of inbreeding is:

a. 0.001 **b. 0.002**

c. 0.005 d. 0.004

110. Which of following exotic breed of cattle is recommended for crossbreeding in hilly tract:

a. Holstein Friesian **b. Jersey**

c. Brown Swiss d. Ayrshire

111. The optimum improvement in milk yield can be observed with exotic inheritance level of:

a. 1/2 **b. 3/5**

c. 3/4 d. 4/5

112. In which of the following species, formation of inbred lines is easiest:

a. Cattle b. Sheep

c. Pigs **d. Poultry**

113. The ONBS utilizes the technology of:

a. Embryo transfer b. Cloning

c. Transgenesis d. PCR

114. The selection of males with ONBS is:

a. Faster **b. Accurate**

c. Real d. Ideal

115. In ONBS, the high milk yielder may be used as:

a. Donor b. Recipient

c. Both of the above d. None of the above

116. The first embryo transfer calf in India was produced in:

a. 1976 **b. 1987**

c. 1992 d. 1998

117. The genetic consequences of inbreeding is:

a. Increase homozygosity b. Increase heterozygosity

c. Increase fertility d. Increase infertility

118. Inbreeding is the mating individuals:

a. Unrelated animals of same breed

b. Related animals of same breed

c. Unrelated animals of different breed

d. Related animals of different breed

119. Karan Swiss and Karan Fries cattle strain were produced by:

a. Inbreeding **b. Cross breeding**

c. Top crossing d. Grading up

120. The increased level of performance of crossbred as compared to the best of parent breed is known as:

a. Heterosis **b. Hybrid vigour**

c. Assortative mating d. Top-crossing

121. Which is most useful when the outstanding individual is dead or not available for breeding purpose:

a. Line breeding b. Out breeding

c. Top crossing d. Back crossing

122. The inbreeding coefficient for half sib mating is:

a. 0.219 **b. 0.125**

c. 0.50 d. 0.3125

123. The relationship coefficient between half sib will be:

a. 0.25 b. 0.125

c. 0.50 d. 0.37

124. Offspring produced by crossing of a male horse (stallion) and female donkey (jenny) is

a. Mule b. Cattalo

c. Hinny d. Jenney

125. The production of mule is result of:

a. Top crossing b. Criss crossing

c. Inbreeding **d. Species hybridization**

126. Heterozygote superiority is due to:

a. Pleiotropism b. Multiple gene action

c. Over dominance d. Additive gene action

127. Decline in the performance will be more as a result of inbreeding which is affected greatly by:

a. Additive gene action **b. Non-additive gene action**

c. Multiple allele d. All of the above

128. Coefficient of relationship between double first cousin is:

a. 0.015 **b. 0.25**

c. 1.00 d. None of the above

129. The mating system which increases hetrozygosity in progenies:

a. Inbreeding b. Line breeding

c. Outbreeding d. None of the above

130. When a highly inbred taster line is crossed with large number of individuals as source population, the system is called:

a. Reciprocal recurrent selection **b. Recurrent selection**

c. Both of the above d. None of the above

131. The new breeds can be evolved by:

a. Criss crossing

b. Reciprocal recurrent selection

c. Cross breeding

d. Out crossinG

132. The method of path coefficient was developed by:

a. Sewall Wright b. J.L.Lush

c. Malecot d. Falconer

133. The generally preferred level of exotic inheritance in crossbreeding programme is:

a. 25% b. 37.5%

c. 50% d. 70%

134. The selection index method for animal application was developed by:

a. Fisher b. Smith

c. Falconer **d. Hazel**

Q.3. Fill in the Blanks

1. The method of path coefficient was given by ***Sewall Wright.***
2. ***Cross breeding*** is the mating of animals from different established breeds.
3. A line can be called close to the inbred line when the coefficient of inbreeding reaches to ***37.5*** percent.
4. ***Coefficient of inbreeding*** of an individual is the probability that the two genes present at a locus are identical by descent.
5. The decrease in performance resulting from inbreeding is called ***inbreeding depression.***
6. Two way flow of genes are possible in ***open nucleus*** scheme.
7. A single population which is a mixture of various populations is called ***synthetic.***
8. After six crosses of purebred sires, the graded animals carry ***98.3*** percent.
9. Parent and offspring mating is an example of ***direct*** relationship.
10. ***Pian niu*** is a cross between cattle and yak.
11. In small population's homozygosity increases due to ***depression*** of genes.
12. Inbreeding leads to genetic ***differentiation*** between lines and genetic ***uniformity with in lines.***
13. Genetic consequence of inbreeding results directly from the increased ***homozygosity.***
14. Commonly used experimental design for crossing the inbred lines is ***Diallel crossing.***
15. The value of coefficient of inbreeding may range from ***0 to 1.0***
16. Three generations of full sib mating would result in an inbreeding coefficient of ***0.5.***
17. The synthetic population will retain ***half*** the total heterosis increment relative to the base population.

18. The consequence of crossbreeding is to increase the ***heterozygosity.***

19. The system of mating used to improve upon a non-descript population to the level of known breed is called ***grading up.***

20. Fitness lost on ***inbreeding*** tends to be restored on ***cross breeding.***

21. The effects of inbreeding will be more on those traits governed by ***non additive effect.***

22. When parents are related to each other more closely than randomly chosen individual, the mating system is called ***inbreeding.***

23. When two breeds are crossed alternatively, the method is ***criss crossing.***

24. The term 'F' to denote inbreeding coefficient was given by ***Wright.***

25. In sheep crossbreeding has been done to improve ***wool quality*** traits.

26. Buffalo breeding policy in India mainly includes ***selective breeding.***

27. Mule is produced by ***species hybridization*** method.

28. ***Line breeding*** is generally practiced to conserve the genes of an outstanding bull.

29. The main genetic effect of inbreeding is ***increased homozygosity.***

30. Sheep breeds of Rajasthan are famous for ***carpet wool.***

31. Average age of individuals when they become parent is known a ***generation interval.***

32. The practical use of inbreeding is to develop ***inbred lines*** that can be used for crossing purpose.

33. Rotational crossing is most suitable for improving ***pigs.***

34. Records of ancestry of animal maintained on farm are called ***pedigree shot.***

35. The minimum number of breeds used in rotational crossbreeding is ***three.***

36. ***Interse*** mating is the system of mating practiced to maintain the inheritance level in crossbred population at a constant level.

37. A progeny produced from cross between mare and male ass (Jack) is known as ***Mule.***

38. Robert Blackwell developed ***Longhorn*** breed of cattle.

39. Degree of genetic relationship between grand sire and daughter is ***25%.***
40. The word/symbol "G means in genetic terms ***genetic gain.***
41. Crossing of non-inbred female population to inbred male is known as ***top crossing.***
42. Mating of unrelated animals within the same pure breed called ***out crossing.***
43. When the average of offspring exceeds the average of their parents the term is known as ***hybrid vigour.***
44. An individual common in pedigree of two individuals is called ***common ancestor.***
45. In crossbreeding, maximum amount of hetrozygosity is achieved in the ***first*** generation.
46. Population derived from crossing of various breed is ***synthetic.***
47. The inbreeding coefficient of an individual resulting from mating of full brothers and full sisters equal to ***25*** percent.
48. Charles & Robert Colling brothers developed the ***shorthorn*** breed of cattle.
49. The relationship of animals with two grand parents in common is ***12.5*** percent.
50. ***Back cross*** is the cross when females are mated to males of one of the parental breed.
51. ***Inbreeding coefficient*** of an individual is the probability that the two genes present at locus are identical by descent.
52. When all individuals are homozygous at all loci the frequency of heterozygotes is ***zero.***
53. Two way flows of genes are possible in ***open nucleus breeding scheme.***
54. The full sibs have the genetic relationship of ***50 percent.***
55. After five crosses of purebred sires, the grade animals carry ***96.9*** percent.
56. ***Fertility*** is very low or nil among the progeny of most species crosses.
57. ***Specific combining ability*** is the ability of two breeds, lines or strains to produce specific effects in progeny when crossed.
58. ONBS is recommended for ***elite*** population.

59. Coefficient of inbreeding of an individual is ***half*** of the coefficient of relationship of its parents.
60. Inbreeding changes ***genotypic*** frequency, not ***gene*** frequency.
61. The number of purebreds used in the rotational crossing is ***2 or 3.***
62. The half sib has the genetic relationship ***25*** percent.
63. The deleterious effects of inbreeding are due to ***homozygosity/uncovering effect***
64. Synonym of random mating is ***Panmixia.***
65. Increased inbreeding is always accompanied by a ***decline*** in fitness trait.
66. Crossbreeding increases ***heterozygosity.***
67. The traits with low heritability are very much affected by ***inbreeding.***
68. The phenomenon where offspring is superior in vigour and performance over the parent is called as ***hybrid vigour***.
69. ***Sannen/Alpine/Anglonubian/Toggenburg*** exotic breeds of goat which have been used in India for crossing purpose.
70. Genetic positive assortative mating is ***inbreeding.***
71. Mating systems affects the distribution of ***genotypes*** in the population.
72. Out crossing followed by selection is very effective for highly ***heritable*** traits.
73. ***Hinny*** is the cross of stallion and jennet.
74. Gene and genotypic frequencies change under ***positive*** assortative mating.
75. Inbreeding ***increases*** variances between lines.
76. There is increase in homozygous genotypes and decrease in heterozygous genotypes due to ***inbreeding.***
77. Small population size lead inevitably to loss of ***heterozygosity.***
78. Inbreeding depression is generally greater for character associated with ***natural fitness.***
79. ***Inbreeding*** affects the extent and distribution of variance and not the mean.
80. Prepotency depends on ***homozygosity.***

81. In random mating population of domestic animals the ***sire/male*** are main contributors to inbreeding coefficient.

82. ***Species hybridization*** is the widest possible kind of out breeding.

83. Progeny of related parents is ***inbred.***

84. Decrease in mean due to inbreeding is because of ***appearance*** of detrimental recessive genes.

85. Disease tolerance is ***polygenically*** inherited.

86. Inbreeding ***decreases*** within line variance and ***increase*** between line variance.

87. The degree of relationship by descent between the two parents is called ***co-ancestery.***

88. For the evaluation of various gene effects ***diallel*** method of analysis is more suitable.

89. For rotational crossing at least ***three*** breeds are needed.

90. For mating system in which all the individuals have equal chance to be parents for the production of offspring for next generation is known a ***random mating.***

91. The progeny of a single individual obtained by selfing is called ***pure line.***

92. The variation within inbred line is more due to ***environmental*** than ***genetic*** causes.

93. Loci without ***dominance*** cause neither inbreeding depression nor heterosis.

94. When heritability for a trait is close to zero, than one should use ***crossbreeding.***

95. Single crossing is mating of a male and female of ***two*** different breeds.

96. Experiments indicate that traits having bearing on fitness are ***depressed*** by inbreeding and show greatest benefit from ***cross breeding.***

97. The coefficient of inbreeding is generally symbolized by ***F.***

98. The system of mating being used for improvement of Indian pigs is ***grading up.***

99. Heterosis is caused by heterozygosity involving genes with ***non-additive*** effects.

100. Different traits of economic importance are affected by both ***additive*** and non-additive gene action.

101. Jersey crosses have better ***reproductive efficiency*** than Friesian crosses.

102. IBL 80 is a strain of ***broiler*** produced in India.

103. Inbred lines play an important role in breeding programme of ***poultry.***

104. The inbreeding coefficient of an individual after three generations of full sib mating will be ***0.5.***

105. Maximum milk in India is obtained from ***buffalo.***

106. A species is ***polytypic*** if composed of genetically distinct breeding population.

107. ***Selfing*** is the most extreme form of inbreeding.

108. Karan swiss breed of cattle was developed at ***NDRI.***

109. ***Rotational crossing*** is the common mating system followed in pigs.

110. Pedigree in which data to indicate the phenotypic merit of ancestors are being included, these pedigree called ***performance pedigrees.***

111. ***System of breeding*** and ***selection*** constitute the only tool available to the breeder for improvement of animals.

112. Extreme form of out breeding is called ***species hybridization.***

113. Seed stock producing herds will follow the mating of ***closely related individuals.***

114. ***Inbreeding*** makes desirable and undesirable genes homozygous impartially.

115. The full form of ONBS is ***Open Nucleus Breeding System.***

116. The inbreeding depression depends on the ***level of dominance.***

117. In ***grading up*** sire of pure breed is mated with a non-descript female.

118. The ability of two or more breeds to combine well to produce superior crossbred offspring is known as ***breed complementation.***

119. The result of crossbreeding is increased due to hetrozygosity.

120. ***Out crossing*** is the mating of unrelated animals within a breed.

121. Least variable trait is ***gestation length.***

122. The coefficient of inbreeding after three generations of half sib mating is ***0.304.***

123. Mating of males and females according to phenotypic likeness is called ***Assortative mating***

124. Inbred parents are more likely to be ***prepotent*** than non inbred parent at least for trait conditioned by dominant gene.

4

Animal Genetics and Breeding: Principles of Animal Breeding

Q.1. True & False

1. False — Progeny testing in dairy cattle takes less time to obtain the results.
2. True — Truncation type selection is usually observed in large populations.
3. False — Milk and fat percentage are positively correlated.
4. False — Carcass traits have low heritability.
5. False — Malvi is a good milch breed of cattle.
6. True — Khaki Campbell and Indian Runner are important egg producing breed of ducks.
7. False — Mehsana is a buffalo breed of Maharashtra state.
8. True — Repeatability is an upper limit of heritability.
9. True — BLUP method can be used to estimate the breeding value of a sire.
10. True — Within family, selection is useful when common environmental effects are important.
11. False — Frieswal cattle have been developed by crossing between HF and Gir.
12. False — Barbari goat is a good milker highly prolific and generally gives birth to triplets.

13. True — India is having highest buffalo population in the world.
14. False — Repeatability estimates of a trait are generally smaller than heritability estimates.
15. True — Phenotypic covariance is the sum of genetic and environmental covariance.
16. True — The principle of progeny testing comes from sampling nature of inheritance.
17. False — The generation interval is the average age of the individual when they become sexually mature.
18. True — The response to selection can be improved by increasing heritability and proportion of individual to be selected.
19. True — In sib selection, the selected individuals do not contribute to the future generation.
20. True — Recurrent selection is one of the important methods of selection to improve both general and specific combining ability of two specific populations regardless of the level of dominance.
21. False — Reciprocal recurrent selection is widely applicable to cattle and other bovines
22. True — Selection for or against a recessive gene is extremely ineffective when the recessive gene is rare.
23. True — India ranks first among the countries of the world in goat population.
24. True — The effect of environment on qualitative characters is negligible.
25. False — The genetic constitution of a population is constant from generation to generation.
26. True — Murrah is the best milk producing breed of buffalo.
27. True — The native tract of Sahiwal cattle is in Pakistan.
28. False — Mandya sheep is famous for fine wool.
29. False — Maximum population of goat is in the state of Rajasthan.
30. True — In U.P. the population of buffalo is increasing at the cost of cattle.

31. True — South Indian sheep breeds are mainly mutton type breed.
32. False — Shahabadi sheep are found in U.P.
33. True — Most of the Indian cattle population is non-descript.
34. True — India ranks first in total milk production in the world.
35. False — The ICL method of selection gives due weightage to h^2 of the trait.
36. True — Selection increases the h^2 of a trait.
37. True — Heritability of a trait is used in estimation of MPPA.
38. True — The reproduction fitness of favoured genotype is generally taken as one.
39. True — Faster genetic progress is possible in multiparous animals.
40. True — Krishnan's index was first sire index proposed in India.
41. True — The intensity of selection is higher in males than females.
42. False — Indian breed of cattle are reputed for their high milk production.
43. False — Gir is the recognized cattle breed of Madhya Pradesh.
44. True — Heritability ranges from 0 to 1.
45. False — Repeatability is used to predict performance of future progeny of an animal.
46. True — No new genes can be created by selection.
47. True — Heritability estimates for productive traits are low.
48. False — Individual selection should predict if the trait is highly heritable.
49. False — Heterozygotes breed true.
50. True — Maximum hetrozygosity is attained in F_1 generation.
51. False — Selection increases genetic variability in a population by creating new genes.
52. False — Artificial selection and natural selection operate simultaneously.
53. True — Within family selection means that all the members of better family are selected.
54. True — Heritability of a trait is particular to a population.

55. False — For highly heritable traits selection should be based on progeny performance.

56. False — Selection reduces mean and increases variation.

57. False — Selection intensity does not depend upon the proportion of selected individual.

58. True — Broad breasted large white turkey was developed from a cross of broad breasted bronze and white Holland breed.

59. True — Berkshire is a known breed of swine.

60. True — Muscovy duck is a meat type breed.

61. False — For sex-linked traits individual selection is used.

62. True — For high heritable traits selection on phenotypic performance is most efficient.

63. False — Genetic response in a trait due to selection is equal to heritability.

64. False — Heritability of any trait cannot be improved by reducing environmental deviations.

65. False — The heritability estimated by regression method is multiplied by four.

66. False — Intensity of selection is more when population retained is large.

67. True — Individual selection yields rapid progress when the heritability of the trait is high.

68. False — Progeny testing is the most valuable aid for selection of traits of high heritability.

69. False — Shorter generation interval always increases genetic progress per year as compared to large generation interval.

70. False — The sire evaluation method by daughter-dam comparison takes care of the confounding effect of environmental variations.

71. False — The basic effect of selection is to change genotypic frequencies.

72. True — Paternal half sib's method is most widely used to determine heritability in farm animals.

73. False — Most traits of economic importance in animal breeding are qualitative in nature.

74. True — The accuracy of individual selection is increased by combining information on family.

75. True — Mass selection is effective for traits with high heritability and expressed earlier in life.

76. True — Simultaneous selection for several characters is superior to selection for single trait at a time to improve the overall merit of the population under selection.

77. False — Maximum fat percent is reported in the milk of murrah breed of buffalo.

78. False — Sib testing and progeny testing are synonyms.

79. True — The genotype remains constant for an animal through out its life.

80. False — Heritability estimated for fitness traits is high in magnitude.

81. True — Repeatability of a trait forms upper limit of heritability estimate of same trait.

82. False — Mandya is pure Indian sheep with lowest medullation percentage.

83. False — Selection can create new genes.

84. False — The response to selection depends upon the repeatability of the trait and the selection differential.

85. True — Gir is the popular cattle breed of Gujarat.

86. True — Regression of breeding value on phenotypic value gives the estimate of heritability.

87. True — If generation interval is larger, genetic progress will be low.

88. True — Barbari breed of goat is most suitable for stall rearing while Black Bengal for high prolificacy.

89. True — Index selection is most effective when number of trait considered are more.

90. True — Traits with low heritability should be given more emphasis in selection index.

91.	True	Repeatability estimates are higher, if numbers of records considered are more.
92.	True	Selection is a relatively slow process of animal improvement.
93.	False	If environmental variations are more, the heritability estimates will be higher.
94.	True	Independent culling level method can be used for selecting more than one trait at a time.
95.	False	When a bull is selected on the basis of his progeny performance it is called individual selection.
96.	True	Variance is always positive.
97.	False	h^2 x SD is formula to get genetic gain per year.
98.	False	Top crossing is extreme form of out breeding.
99.	False	Murrah is an endangered breed of buffalo.
100.	True	The generation interval in Indian cattle is about 5 years.
101.	False	The h^2 estimate will be 0.2 when regression of offspring on mid parent is 0.4.
102.	True	The genetic correlation is the correlation of breeding values.
103.	True	Recurrent selection is method for utilizing specific combining ability.
104.	True	Muzaffarnagri is a heaviest Indian breed of sheep.
105.	True	South Indian sheep breeds are known for mutton production.
106.	False	Repeatability and heritability are used in selection indices.
107.	True	Reciprocal recurrent selection in poultry was first suggested by Bell.
108.	False	J.L.Lush is known as the father of animal breeding.
109.	False	White Leghorn is a rose comb breed.
110.	True	The colour of Sirohi breed of goat is brown.
111.	True	Most of the economic traits in domestic animals are quantitative.
112.	False	A trait might be influenced by a gene.

113. True — All non-genetic influences are usually considered together as environment.

114. False — Environment is defined as comparing all influences apart of additive effects.

115. False — Observed phenotypic variance is caused by different genotypes of groups of animals.

116. True — If there are no genotype-environmental interactions, the phenotypic variance is the combination of genotypic and environmental variance.

117. True — The real producing ability or performance potential of an animal is estimated by following equation P=b(O-M)+M.

118. False — The temporary effects are independent from period to period and they are likely to be positive.

119. True — The coefficient of heritability is not constant but only indicates the proportion of variance caused by differences in additive gene effects in a particular population at a particular time.

120. True — The genetic correlation between two traits is the correlation between gene effects influencing them.

121. True — Genetic correlation is caused mostly by pleiotropy.

122. False — To breeders progress per year is not important than progress per generation.

123. True — The herd book system was first introduced to provide information on ancestors.

124. True — Progeny testing means taking the performance of offspring as the criterion for selection among the parents.

125. True — Heritability cannot be more than repeatability.

126. True — Toggenburg is a known milch breed of goat.

127. False — Genetic and phenotypic correlation are always in same direction.

128. False — Sire index phenotypic correlation is always genetic principles.

129. True — Reciprocal recurrent selection is effective in low heritability traits.

130. False — Difference between means of sire and dam is called as selection differential.

131. True — Selection is the choosing of parents for next generation.

132. True — *Bos taurus* is the name given to exotic cattle.

133. False — Family selection is preferred when character has high heritability.

134. False — General combining ability of a genotype is due to non-additive effects of the genes.

135. False — In contemporary comparison method of progeny testing, age correction are required.

136. True — Breeder can maximize genetic gain by reducing generation interval.

137. False — In reciprocal recurrent selection source population is crossed with tester population.

138. True — The range of correlation is -1 to+1.

139. True — Duck eggs are15-20 gm heavier than the chicken egg.

140. True — Anglo-Nubian is known as the jersey cow of the goat world.

141. False — Mass selection is best suited for sex limited traits.

142. True — Excellent herd of Kankrej breed of cattle are found in Brazil.

143. True — In reciprocal recurrent selection two source populations are crossed reciprocally.

144. False — Specific combining ability is due to additive gene action.

145. False — Barbari is the breed of goat in India which gives maximum number of kids.

146. True — Planning of any breeding programme requires prior knowledge of genetic parameters.

147. True — Milk yield and fat yield are negatively correlated.

148. True — Selection does not create new genes.

149. True — The fat percentage of Bhadawari buffalo is higher than Murrah.

150. False — Collateral relatives are the individual sire, dam, grand sire and grand dam.

151. False — Heritability of a trait does not vary from time to time.

152. False — Tandem selection is superior to independent culling level selection.

153. True — General combining ability is due to the additive effect of genes and additive x additive interaction.

154. True — Inbreeding increases the homozygosity of both the desirable and undesirable genes.

155. True — Aseel breed of poultry is famous for its majestic gait and dog fighting qualities.

156. False — Information on relatives is important for selection when h^2 of the trait is high.

157. True — Jersey is the exotic dairy cattle breed preferred for its adaptability and higher fat percentage.

158. False — Pedigree selection is better than progeny testing.

159. False — Southdown is a popular fine wool breed of sheep.

160. False — Selection index and sire index are synonyms.

161. True — A correlated response is the change in an unselected trait resulting from selection of another trait.

162. True — Operating system controls all the functions being performed on the hard disk and controls all the instructions given to the computer.

Q.2. Multiple Choices :

1. The selection index method for animal application was developed by:

   a. R.A. Fisher — b. Smith

   c. Falconer — **d. Hazel**

2. In poultry the character of low heritability is:

   a. Egg production — b. Egg weight

   c. Fertility — d. None of the above

3. The good milch breed of cattle is:

   a. Red Sindhi — b. Nimari

   c. Hallikar — d. None of the above

4. Corrected daughter average index was given by:

   a. Edwards — b. Hanson

   c. Krishnan — d. Jain and Malhotra

5. Heritability estimated by half sib intraclass correlation measures:

   a. ½ VA + ¼ VA + 1/16 VA

   b. 1/8 VA + 1/16 VA + 1/64 VA

   c. ¼ VA + 1/16 VA + __

   d. None of the above

6. Selection index method is superior to:

   a. Tandem method b. Independent culling method

   c. Both of the above d. None of the above

7. The minimum number of daughters required to achieve 80% accuracy of selection in progeny testing for milk yield are:

   a. 5 b. 10

   c. 22 d. None of the above

8. Karakul breed of sheep is important for:

   a. Wool production b. Fur production

   c. Pelt production d. None of the above

9. Anglo-Nubian is an important breed of goat for:

   a. Mutton production **b. Milk production**

   c. Both of the above d. None of the above

10. Accuracy of selection is the:

    a. Correlation between breeding value and phenotypic value

    b. Regression of breeding value on phenotypic value

    c. Both of the above d. None of the above

11. National Bureau of Animal Genetic Resources is located at:

    a. Hissar b. Ludhiana

    c. Karnal d. None of the above

12. Selection on the basis of individuality is most important when h^2 of the trait is:

    a. Low b. Medium

    c. High d. None of the above

13. Exotic breed of goat is:

a. Barbari **b. Sannen**

c. Surti d. None of the above

14. Accuracy of selection in individual selection when based on single record equals:

a. H^2 b. ½ h^2

c. ¼ h^2 d. h

15. Breed of poultry famous for its magestic gait and dog fighting qualities is:

a. Kadaknath **b. Aseel**

c. Punjab brown d. None of the above

16. Tamworth, Large White Yorkshire and Berkshire breeds were imported from:

a. England b. U.S.A.

c. Canada d. Japan

17. The regression of breeding value on phenotypic value provide estimate of:

a. Repeatability **b. Heritability**

c. Correlated response d. None of the above

18. The permanent cause of genetic correlation between two lines is due to:

a. Linkage **b. Pleiotropy**

c. Both of the above d. None of the above

19. The least efficient method of selection is:

a. Tandem method b. Independent culling method

c. Selection index d. Individual selection

20. A record of an individual ancestors who are related to him through his parents is known as:

a. Family selection b. Mass selection

c. Progeny testing d. Pedigree

21. When the heritability of a trait is high, the best selection procedure to improve the population is:

    a. Family selection
    b. Sib selection
    c. Individual selection
    d. None of the above

22. In recurrent selection the tester line is usually:

    a. An inbred line
    b. Open bred line
    c. Both of the above
    d. None of the above

23. Selection can be intensified if population size is:

    a. Increased
    b. Decreased
    c. Constant
    d. None of the above

24. Fur type wool is produced by one of the following breed of sheep:

    a. Karakul
    b. Gurej
    c. Bhakarwal
    d. Gaddi

25. Precision of the heritability estimate depends on its:

    a. Standard error
    b. Coefficient of variation
    c. Sampling variance
    d. All of the above

26. Selection based on the performance of the individual, its full sibs and half sibs is known as:

    a. Family selection
    b. Sire family selection
    c. Combined selection
    d. None of the above

27. Selection of animals for improvement in one set of condition would also result in genetic improvement in another in absence of:

    a. Genetic variation
    b. Environmental variation
    c. Genotypic environmental interaction
    d. None of the above

28. Generation interval is likely to be prolonged when selection is based on:

    a. Life time performance of an individual
    b. Pedigree performance
    c. Progeny performance
    d. Collateral relatives performance

29. Which of the following is small sized breed of goat:

    a. Jamunapari b. Beetal

    c. Black Bengal d. Sirohi

30. The latest method of sire evaluation is:

    a. Equal parent index b. Rice index

    c. Krishnan's index **d. BLUP**

31. The father of selective livestock breeding is:

    a. Robert Bakewell b. Lush

    c. Wright d. Rice

32. Which of the following is not a wild relative of cattle:

    a. Gaur b. Gayal

    c. Yak **d. Zebu**

33. Which of the following breeds have not contributed for developing "Karan Swiss" breed of cattle:

    a. Sahiwal b. Red Sindhi

    c. Holstein Friesian d. Brown Swiss

34. Which of the following is most endangered breed of buffalo:

    a. Murrah b. Nili Ravi

    c. Bhadawari d. Mehsana

35. Jhakrana breed of goat is famous in:

    a. U.P. b. Rajasthan

    c. Haryana d. Punjab

36. In Rajasthan, number of sheep breeds is:

    a. 6 **b. 8**

    c. 16 d. 18

37. The simultaneous improvement in many traits can be obtained by using:

    a. Mass selection **b. Inclepent culling levels**

    c. Selection index d. None of the above

38. The selection differential depends on:
    a. Phenotypic variability
    b. Proportion of selected individual
    c. Both of the above
    d. None of the above
39. Which of the following parameter is used in estimation of response to selection:
    a. Heritability
    b. Repeatability
    c. Genetic correlation
    d. None of the above
40. If h^2 of milk yield is 0.3 and selection differential of selected cows is 300kg, the expected genetic response will be:
    a. 90 kg
    b. 45 kg
    c. 180 kg
    d. 300 kg
41. The constants needed to construct the selection index may be:
    a. H^2
    b. Genetic correlation
    c. Economic value
    d. All of the above
42. Genetic gain per unit time can be calculated by using:
    a. Generation interval
    b. Phenotypic mean
    c. Breeding value
    d. None of the above
43. Actual genetic worth of an animal is judged on the basis of its:
    a. Own performance
    b. Pedigree performance
    c. Sib's performance
    d. Progeny performance
44. Half-sib individuals are those having:
    a. Common sire and different dams
    b. Both sires and dams are common
    c. Both sires and dams are different
    d. None of the above
45. Estimation of heritability from regression of offspring on dam equals:
    a. 2×boS
    b. 2×boD
    c. boP
    d. None of the above

46. In crossing inbred lines where each line is crossed with every other line is called:

    a. Top crossing
    b. Diallel crossing
    c. RPS
    d. None of the above

47. The most important distribution encounterd in biological date is:

    a. Passon
    b. Normal
    c. Binomial
    d. None of the above

48. Sib selection is different from family selection in that:

    a. The selected individuals are measured
    b. The selected individuals are not measured
    c. Only males are measured
    d. Only females are measured

49. In poultry a character of low h^2 is:

    a. Egg production
    b. Egg weight
    c. Fertility
    d. None of the above

50. Sunandini is a breed of cattle developed in:

    a. Karnal
    b. West Bengal
    c. Kerala
    d. Gujrat

51. Jaffarabadi is buffalo breed of :

    a. Madhya Pradesh
    b. Maharashtra
    c. Gujarat
    d. Karnataka

52. Specific combining ability is due to:

    a. Additive gene action
    b. Polygenic
    c. Non-additive gene action
    d. None of the above

53. Corrected daughter average index was given by:

    a. Edwards
    b. Hansson
    c. Krishnan
    d. Jain and Malhotra

54. Long pendulous ears and roman nose are the characteristic of following goat breed:

a. Barbari
b. Osmanabadi
c. Jamunapari
d. Beetal

55. The Leghorn fowl belongs to the class:

a. American
b. Mediterranean
c. English
d. Asiatic

56. Popular buffalo breed from Saurashtra region of Gujrat is:

a. Mehsana
b. Jaffarabadi
c. Murrah
d. None of the above

57. Selection is more effective when:

a. There is more uniformity among animals
b. There is more genetic variability in the population
c. Individuals are alike
d. None of the above

58. Measure of regression of future performance on past performance is called :

a. Heritability
b. Repeatability
c. Selection intensity
d. None of the above

59. Selection differential is a:

a. Difference of progeny mean and population mean
b. Superiority of the progeny
c. Superiority of the selected parents over the population mean
d. None of the above

60. Selection index method is superior to:

a. Tandem method
b. Independent culling level
c. Both of the above
d. None of the above

61. Estimation of heritability by full sib correlation method equals:

a. 4t
b. 2t
c. t
d. None of the above

62. A main cause of genetic correlation between two trait is:

a. Genetic polymorphism **b. Genetic pleiotropy**

c. Hetrozygosity d. Non genetic inheritance

63. The estimation of heritability based on selection experiments is called:

a. Narrow sense h^2 b. Broad sense h^2

c. Realised h^2 d. None of the above

64. The origin of Landrace breed of pig is from:

a. England b. Poland

c. Denmark d. None of the above

65. The two main important egg producing breeds of duck are:

a. Khaki Campbell and Orpington

b. Indian runner and Orpington

c. Khaki Campbell and Indian Runner

d. None of the above

66. The most prolific Indian goat breed is:

a. Barbari b. Jamunapari

c. Black Bengal d. Beetal

67. Prominent draught cattle breed with its home tract in Mysore region is:

a. Dangi **b. Hallikar**

c. Kangayam d. Khillari

68. Which of the following is a layer breed:

a. Aseel b. Kadaknath

c. Cornish **d. White Leghorn**

69. The result of progeny testing is expressed in terms of:

a. Selection index **b. Sire index**

c. Sex index d. Regression

70. Response to selection divided by selection differential gives estimate of:

a. Heritability **b. Realized heritability**

c. Repeatability d. Breeding value

71. When heritability of the traits is high, the best basis of selection will be:

    a. Mass selection b. Family selection

    c. Progeny testing d. Index selection

72. Tandem method of selection is used for genetic improvement of traits which are:

    a. Negatively related b. Skewed type

    c. Independent traits d. Bimodal traits

73. Selection differential will be maximum in a trait having:

    a. High heritability b. High genetic variance

    c. High phenotypic variance d. High non-genetic variance

74. Breeders can increase genetic gain per year by reducing:

    a. Heritability b. Selection differential

    c. Repeatability **d. Generation interval**

75. When two traits are negatively correlated, improvements in one trait lead to:

    a. Decline in other trait b. Increase in other unit

    c. No effect on other trait d. None of the above

76. The main utility of chegu breed of goat is for the production of:

    a. Meat **b. Pashmina**

    c. Milk d. Hair

77. Recurrent selection exploits:

    a. Additive gene action **b. Non-additive gene action**

    c. Both a & b d. None of the above

78. Traits of economic importance in livestock are:

    a. Quantitative traits b. Qualitative traits

    c. Both a & b d. None of the above

79. Heritability is the ratio of:
    a. Genotypic and environmental variances
    b. Genotypic and additive genetic variances
    c. Additive genetic and environmental variances
    d. None of the above
80. Selection differential is:
    a. Superiority of selected parents over the population mean
    b. Superiority of the progeny
    c. Difference of progeny mean and population mean
    d. None of the above
81. Selection refers to:
    a. Allowing superior animals to reproduce
    b. Rejecting inferior animals
    c. Both a & b
    d. None of the above
82. Selection for additive gene action is named as:
    a. Intrapopulation selection
    b. Interpopulation selection
    c. Reciprocal recurrent selection
    d. Recurrent selection
83. Natural selection becomes operative when new genetic variations are created through:
    a. Mutation
    b. Migration
    c. Isolation due to geographic reasons
    d. All of the above
84. Selection and culling:
    a. Operate simultaneously
    b. Are opposite of each other
    c. Are pre-requisite of each other
    d. All of the above

85. In directional selection individuals are selected whose phenotype approach have:

    a. Maximum value b. Intermediate value

    c. Near to mean d. None of the above

86. Most important factor responsible for improvement is:

    a. Genetic interval **b. Heritability**

    c. Choice of environment d. Growth rate

87. Intrasire regression of offspring on dam estimates:

    a. Heritability b. Repeatability

    c. Half the heritability d. One fourth heritability

88. The family selection is the method of choice for traits with:

    a. Low heritability b. High heritability

    c. Expression in one sex only d. Large family size

89. When selection is practiced for two or more traits at a time and for each trait a minimum standard is set. The method of selection used is called:

    a. Tandem method **b. Independent culling method**

    c. Progeny testing method d. Selection index method

90. Recurrent selection method is recommended when there is significant:

    a. Over dominance

    b. Dominance

    c. Epistasis

    d. Overdominance cum epistasis

91. Suffolk and Dorset are the exotic breed of sheep which may be used in India for improvement of:

    a. Wool b. Milk

    c. Pelt **d. Mutton production**

92. When the character is measured of the individual after its death then method of selection used is:

    a. Individual selection b. Mass selection

    c. Sib selection d. None of the above

93. Progeny testing is a method of selection where in:

  a. Selection of the individual is based on the offspring's performance

  b. Selection of the progeny is on the basis of their mean phenotypic value

  c. Selection of outstanding progeny after testing them

  d. Selection of progeny of a sire, after comparison with their contemporaries

94. When response to selection has ceased, the population is said to be at the:

  a. Zero response b. Response limit

  c. Selection limit d. No response

95. Term selection is meant choosing of individual:

  a. To be used as parent for the next generation

  b. Above the population means

  c. Genetically superior

  d. Phenotipically superior

96. A superior and practical evaluation method for sires:

  a. Herd mate daughter comparison

  b. Pedigree comparison

  c. Dam-daughter comparison

  d. Daughter average (100)

97. The difference between the mean phenotypic values of the selected individuals from the mean of the entire population before selection is called as:

  a. Response to selection **b. Selection differential**

  c. Genetic gain d. Genetic advance

98. Best estimate of an individuals breeding value to act as a basis of selection is:

  a. Performance of its progeny b. Pedigree performance

  c. Individuals own performance d. Family performance

99. With advent of computer facilities when breeder is interested in progress of several economic traits, the selection method of choice is:

a. Independent culling b. Tandem selection

c. Random selection **d. Index selection**

100. The index selection is efficient over other methods of selection because its takes account of:

a. Heritability of the traits

b. Relative economic weights of the trait

c. Genetic and phenotypic correlation between the traits

d. All of the above

101. Embryo transfer involves:

a. Super ovulation of the donor

b. Synchronization of both donor and recipient

c. All of the above

d. None of the above

102. Generation interval in cattle is of:

a. 1-2 years **b. 3-4 years**

c. 6-7 years d. 8-10 years

103. Individuals of a breed usually have:

a. Different geographical distribution

b. Common descent

c. Different body characteristic

d. Different production performance

104. Most of Indian buffaloes are of:

a. Swamp type **b. Reverine type**

c. Both swamp and reverine d. None of the above

105. Indian breeds of cattle are reputed for their:

a. Low heat tolerance

b. High milk production

c. High disease resistance

d. Inability to thrive on coarse feeds

106. Contemporary comparison method is used for estimation of:

a. Selection index **b. Sire index**

c. Sex index d. Heterosis

107. Angus is the breed of:

a. Diary cow **b. Beef cattle**

c. Fine wool sheep d. Exotic milk goat

108. White strips around the jaws and brisket is the peculiarity of (buffalo):

a. Jaffarabadi **b. Surti**

c. Mehsana d. Nagpuri breed

109. Primary effect of selection in a population is to:

a. Maintain the population mean

b. Decrease heterozygosity

c. Increase the gene frequency of desirable trait

d. Increase homozygosity

110. In half-sib correlation method of h^2 estimation the intraclass correlation (t) is multiplied by:

a. 4 b. 3

c. 2 d. 8

111. Which goat breed is predominantly found in UP:

a. Black Bengal b. Beetal

c. Jamunapari d. Pashmina

112. Major cause of genetic correlation is:

a. Dominance b. Epistasis

c. Pleiotropy d. Polymorphism

113. Expected genetic gain per year depends on:

a. Repeatbility
b. Sire index
c. Generation interval
d. Correlation

114. Sire index is a numerical score assigned to estimates its:

a. Economic value
b. Selective value
c. Breeding value
d. Adaptive value

115. Indian poultry breed includes:

a. White leghorn
b. Cornish
c. Kadaknath
d. Polymotuh rock

116. Low h^2 estimate is observed from the characters associated with:

a. Carcass trait
b. Reproductive fitness
c. Production traits
d. All of the above

117. Hinny was produced by:

a. Crossbreeding
b. Grading up
c. Out crossing
d. Species hybridization

118. The expected response under individual selection is:

a. $16ph^2$
b. $16p^2h^2$
c. $16p^2h$
d. $16fh^2f$

119. A group of individuals which have certain common characters that distinguish from other group of individuals are called:

a. Individual
b. Breed
c. Species
d. None of the above

120. Which of the following is not a breed of buffalo:

a. Murrah
b. Nili Ravi
c. Nali
d. Bhadawari

121. Which one of the following breed of goat produces maximum milk:

a. Beetal
b. Barbari
c. Jamunapari
d. Black Bengal

122. Reciprocal recurrent selection has no practical use in:

a. Cattle | b. Buffalo
c. Camel | **d. All of the above**

123. Non-random differential reproduction of genotypes is:

a. Selection | b. Selection differential
c. Selection coefficient | d. Fitness

124. The easiest method of estimating heritability of a trait in poultry is:

a. Half sib analysis | **b. Full sib analysis**
c. Twin analysis | d. Regression

125. The home tract of Jamnapari goat is:

a. U.P. | b. Rajaasthan
c. Bihar | d. Orissa

126. Bacterian camel is found in:

a. Rajasthan | **b. Laddakh**
c. Arunachal Pradesh | d. Nagaland

127. Which of the following species has no specific breed in India:

a. Horse | **b. Pig**
c. Camel | d. Cattle

128. Yaks are employed for:

a. Draught | b. Milk
c. Meat | **d. All of the above**

129. Which of the sire evaluation method is suitable in India for genetic evaluation of bulls:

a. BLUP | b. CC
c. Krishnan's index | d. Tomar's index

130. The heritability of milk production is generally:

a. Low | **b. Medium**
c. Moderate | d. High

131. Repeatability is the upper limit of:

a.	Genetic correlation	**b.**	**Heritability**
c.	MPPA	d.	Sire index

132. Selection of cows is generally done by:

a.	Mass selection	b.	ICL
c.	**Index selection**	d.	None of the above

133. Heritability of milk yield in cattle and buffalo is generally estimated by:

a.	**Half sib analysis**	b.	Twin analysis
c.	Full sib analysis	d.	None of the above

134. Identify the scientist concerned with animal breeding:

a.	**Lush**	b.	Newton
c.	Khurana	d.	Watson

135. Tharparkar is a cattle breed found in:

a.	Maharashtra	b.	Kerala
c.	**Rajasthan**	d.	Goa

136. Landrace is an exotic breed of:

a.	**Pig**	b.	Cattle
c.	Poultry	d.	Goat

137. Identity the dual purpose breed of cattle:

a.	**Kankrej**	b.	Kangayam
c.	Hallikar	d.	Malvi

138. National research center on camel is located at:

a.	Pantnagar	b.	Hissar
c.	**Bikaner**	d.	Karnal

139. Kangayam and Hallikar are:

a.	Good milker	**b.**	**Draught animals**
c.	Beef animals	d.	Both a & b

140. In which of the following method of selection a minimum standard is fixed to each traits for selection:

a. Tandem method
b. Selection index
c. Progeny testing
d. Independent culling method

141. Progeny tests may be used in selection for which traits:

a. Qualitative only
b. Quantitative only
c. Both a & b
d. None of the above

142. When h^2 of a character is low, the best method of selection is:

a. Tandem method
b. Selection index
c. Independent culling method
d. None of the above

143. While crossing offspring and mid parent, the h^2 value of a character is measured as:

a. $h^2=b$
b. $h^2=2b$
c. $h^2=4t$
d. $h^2=b^2$

144. General combining ability is due to:

a. Additive gene action
b. Epistasis
c. Over dominance
d. None of the above

145. Which of the sheep breed may be considered as ideal carpet wool:

a. Magra
b. Marwari
c. Chokla
d. Nali

146. Survibility is having:

a. Low h^2
b. Medium h^2
c. High h^2
d. Zero h^2

147. In mule gene action is:

a. Dominant
b. Recessive
c. Over dominance
d. Epistasis

148. Response to selection will be highest for a single trait :

a. Tandem method
b. Total score method
c. Independent culling method
d. None of the above

149. Accuracy of selection based on single record in individual selection equals:

a. 1/2h b. 1/4h

c. 1/8h **d. H**

150. Sib selection is different from selection in that:

a. The selected individuals are measured

b. The selected individuals are not measured

c. Only males are measured

d. Only females are measured

151. Sunandini is a breed of cattle developed in:

a. Karnal b. West Bengal

c. Kerala d. Gujrat

152. Jaffarabadi is buffalo breed of:

a. Madhya Pradesh b. Maharashtra

c. Gujarat d. Karnataka

153. The good milk breed of cattle is:

a. Sahiwal b. Malvi

c. Hariana d. Hallikar

154. Specific combining ability is due to:

a. Additive gene action b. Polygenic

c. Non-additive gene action d. None of the above

155. Heritability estimated by intraclass half-sib correlation measures genetic variation as :

a. ½ VA+1/4VD+1/4AA **b. 1/4 VA+1/16VAA+——**

c. 1/4VA+1/2VD——+ d. None of the above

156. The exotic breeds of cattle used at various centeres of AICRP on cattle are:

a. Jersey and Brown Swiss

b. Brown Swiss & HF

c. Jersey, Brown Swiss and Holstein Friesian

d. HF and Jersey

157. Central Institute for Buffalo Research is located at :

a. Karnal
b. Bangalore
c. Hisar
d. IVRI Izatnagar

158. Accuracy of selection is :

a. Correlation between breeding value and phenotype value
b. Regression of breeding value on phenotype value
c. Both of the above
d. None of the above

159. Estimation of heritability based on selection experiments is called:

a. Narrow sense h^2
b. Broad sense h^2
c. Realised h^2
d. None of the above

160. The repeatability is used to find out :

a. Most probable breeding value
b. Most probable producing ability
c. Realized heritability
d. Regression index

161. Sire index is a numerical score assigned to individual to estimate its:

a. Selective value
b. Economic value
c. Breeding value
d. Generation interval

Q.3. Fill in the Blanks

1. The estimate of h^2 obtained from selection experiments is called **realized h^2**.
2. Full sib family is most common in ***pigs and poultry.***
3. ***Surti*** is a buffalo breed whose horns are sickle shaped.
4. Nimari breed of cattle is an admixture of ***Gir and Khillari*.**
5. When selection differential is expressed in standard deviation units it is known as ***intensity of selection*.**
6. The amount of genetic progress expected depends upon ***h^2SD.***
7. The term heterosis was coined by ***G.H.Shull.***

8. The term MPPA was given by ***J.L.Lush.***
9. The causes of genetic correlation are ***pleiotropy, linkage and hetrozygosity.***
10. Long pendulous ears and Roman nose are the characteristics of ***Jamunapari*** goat.
11. Specific combining ability is due to ***non additive*** gene action.
12. Two new breeds of sheep developed at CSWRI, Avikanagar through crossbreeding are ***Avikalin and Avivastra.***
13. Two new breeds of cattle developed a NDRI, Karnal are ***Karan Swiss and Karan Fries.***
14. An assessment of individual breeding value is based on phenotypic value of ***individual, pedigree, collateral and progeny.***
15. ***Large White Yorkshire*** breed carries the title "The mother breed".
16. Gujrat has three distinct buffalo breeds namely ***Jaffarabadi, Surti and Mehsana.***
17. ***Thaparkar and Hariana*** are dual purpose breeds of cattle.
18. ***Selection*** means choosing of individual to be used as parents.
19. The evaluation of the transmitting ability of an individual by studying the performance of its offspring is ***progeny testing.***
20. Repeatability estimate is the ***intraclass correlation*** among the repeated records of the individual.
21. The reliability of first record as selection criteria for a particular trait depends upon ***repeatability*** estimate of the trait.
22. When several characters have to be selected most suitable method is ***total score method.***
23. The colour of ear lobe is ***white*** in Mediterranean breeds of poultry.
24. The amount of selection pressure applied on a particular trait is known as the ***selection differential.***
25. There are two ways in which the action of the breeder can change the genetic properties of a population. They are ***selection*** and ***breeding.***

26. Simultaneous selection for four traits reduces the selection intensity of any one trait by ***one half.***

27. ***Variation*** is the raw material for the animal breeder with which he has to work for improvement of animals.

28. Independent culling level selection for all the characters is done at the same time but independently rejecting all individuals that fail to come up to a ***minimum*** standard.

29. The BLUP method of sire evaluation was suggested by ***Henderson.***

30. The home tract of Amritmahal breed of cattle is the state of ***Karnataka.***

31. ***Chokla*** breed of sheep is best carpet wool producing bred found in Rajasthan.

32. Chegu goat produces ***Pashmina.***

33. In India, progeny testing of bulls are carried out for mainly improving ***milk production.***

34. Even after cooking the colour of Kadaknath breed of poultry is ***black.***

35. Zanskari and Kathiawari are breeds of ***horse.***

36. ***Breeding value*** determines the value of animals based on mean performance of its progeny.

37. Mass selection is practiced when h^2 of the trait is ***high.***

38. ICL method of selection is used to improve ***more than one*** trait.

39. Differential ***reproduction*** and ***survival*** rate is known as selection.

40. Generally males are selected on the basis of their ***progeny*** performance.

41. In reciprocal recurrent selection two ***divergent*** strains are considered for developing commercial pullets.

42. ***Sire index*** is the numerical value which corresponds to the breeding value of the animal.

43. Black Bengal breed of goat is most ***prolific*** breed.

44. ***Generation interval*** is the average age of parents when their offspring are born.

45. Karan Fries breed of cattle is a cross of ***Thaparkar and Holstein Friesian.***

46. Estimation of heritability based on regression of offspring on mid parent value equals ***bO'P.***

47. Selection on the basis of ancestor's performance is called ***pedigree selection.***

48. Repeatability is a ***higher*** limit of heritability.

49. Angora breed of goat is famous for ***Mohair*** production.

50. Regression of breeding value on phenotypic value gives an estimate that is known as ***heritability.***

51. The value of h^2 ranged from 0 to ***1 or 0 to 100 percent***.

52. The family selection is feasible only in ***prolific*** species.

53. ***Breeding value*** is equal to the sum of average effect of the genes it carries.

54. Hallikar and Amritmahal are important cattle breeds of ***Karnataka state.***

55. National Bureau of Animal Genetic Resources is located at ***Karnal.***

56. Hissardale breed of sheep is a cross of ***Merino×Bikaneri (Magra).***

57. Karakul breed of sheep is important for ***lamb pelt*** production.

58. ***Kadaknath*** is the indigenous breed of poultry in which most of the internal organs are of black colour.

59. The variation exhibited by the quantitative traits is of ***continuous*** type.

60. Genetic gain will be ***zero*** when the h^2 of trait is zero.

61. Breeder can maximize genetic gain/year reducing ***generation interval.***

62. Pleiotropy and ***linkage*** are two important causes of genetic correlation.

63. Selection index method of selection incorporates ***several*** traits.

64. Avikalin and Avivastra are two new breeds of ***sheep.***

65. If generation interval is longer, genetic progress will be ***low/less.***

66. Genetic gain per generation depends on selection differential and ***heritability.***

67. When individuals are selected solely on the basis of phenotypic value, it is called ***mass selection.***

68. The buffalo breed famous for high fat percentage in milk is ***Bhadawari.***

69. Kathiawari is the breed of ***horse.***

70. In-half-sib correlation method of h^2 estimation, the intra-class correlation (t) is multiplied by ***4.***

71. ***Repeatability*** is used to predict future performance of an animal.

72. Standardization of records increases ***accuracy*** of selection.

73. The Indian breed of goat which is most suitable for stall rearing is ***Barbari.***

74. Jamunapari and Beetal goat breeds belong to ***northern-central*** region of India.

75. Merino sheep breed is known for ***fine wool.***

76. Selection is practiced to decrease the frequency of ***undesirable genes.***

77. Breeds of sheep are classified as fine, medium and long on the basis of ***wool*** quality.

78. ***Murrah*** is the best diary breed of buffalo in the world.

79. Corriedale sheep is a ***dual*** purpose breed.

80. ***Sannen*** is known as jersey cow of the goat world.

81. Name one important exotic cattle breed ***Holstein Friesian.***

82. Malabari goat belongs to ***southern*** region of India.

83. Traits linked with profit from animals are called ***economic traits.***

84. ***Directional*** selection is mainly used by animal breeder.

85. ***Hariana*** is a dual purpose breed of cattle of Haryana state.

86. Permanent genetic correlations are caused by ***pleiotropy*** and transient genetic correlation by ***linkage.***

87. The correlation(r) between measurements of the same individual is known as ***repeatability.***

88. Precision of heritability estimate is indicated by its ***standard error.***

89. Tightly curled spiral horn is a typical characteristic of ***Murrah*** buffalo.

90. Holstein breed of cattle is preferred for more ***milk yield*** while Jersey for more ***fat percent.***

91. Name any two breeds of goat famous for pashmina (1) ***Chegu*** and (2) ***Changthangi.***

92. Australorp breed of poultry belongs to ***English*** class.
93. Indian breeds used under All India Coordinated Research Project on cattle were ***Hariana, Ongole*** and ***Gir.***
94. There are ***40*** breeds of sheep and ***20*** breeds of goat in India.
95. Negative phenotypic correlation exists between milk yield and ***butter/fat.***
96. Tandem selection is the selection for each character singly in ***successive*** generations.
97. Selection can act only when there is ***variability.***
98. High heritability indicates a high correlation between ***genotype*** and phenotype.
99. The chief use of measurements of the degree of resemblance between relative is to estimate ***heritability.***
100. MOET stands for ***multiple ovulation and embryo transfer***.
101. ***White Cornish*** is always used as male line parent for better broiler production.
102. Tandem method is useful for ***single*** trait(s).
103. Mass selection is useful for trait with ***high*** heritability estimate.
104. ***Black Bengal*** is the breed of goat (India) which gives maximum number of kids/kidding.
105. Selection differential is inversely proportional to percentage of population ***selected.***
106. Popular buffalo breed from Saurastra region of Gujarat state is ***Mehsana.***
107. For estimation of most probable proucing ability (MPPA), the important parameter needed is ***repeatability.***
108. A system of cross breeding which systematically uses three or more breed is known is ***rotational*** breeding.
109. ***Bhadawari*** breed of buffaloes is known for its high percentage of fat in milk.
110. Toggenburg is a known ***milk*** breed of ***goat.***
111. Sire index express the ***breeding value*** of a bull.

112. Highest milk producing breed of cattle in the world is ***Holstein Friesian.***

113. Mohair is produced by ***Angora*** goat.

114. Individual selection is practiced when correlation between genotype and phenotype is ***one or closer to one.***

115. The primary effect of selection for a character is to change the ***population mean.***

116. The main organization in India for conducting research on MOET is ***NDDB.***

117. Karan Swiss is a newly developed breed of ***cattle.***

118. ***Pigs*** are known to be most prolific specific species among domestic animals.

119. Maximum poultry production in India is in the state of ***Andhra Pradesh.***

120. When the response of selection has ceased, the population is said to be at ***selection plateau.***

121. Genetic gain per unit time depends on ***generation interval.***

122. The rate at which genetic progress can be made depends upon ***heritability.***

123. In reciprocal recurrent selection we use two ***divergent*** populations.

124. The selection index is the best linear prediction of an individual's ***breeding value.***

125. ***White Leghorn*** is the best layer breed in the in world.

126. The combined selection is expected to give ***better*** response than individual selection.

127. The range of heritability lies between ***zero*** to ***one.***

128. ***Kankrej*** breed of cattle is known for its beautiful gait (Sawai chal).

129. The value of an individual judged by the mean value of its progeny is called the ***breeding value*** of that individual.

130. Black Bengal is an indigenous ***meat*** breed of goat whereas Jamunapari is an indigenous ***milk*** breed of goat.

131. Heritability of reproductive traits is very ***low.***

132. ***Repeatability estimates*** are the fraction of differences between single records of individuals that is likely to occur in future records of those same two individuals.

133. The ratio of response to selection differential is ***realized heritability.***

134. The genetic covariance of offspring and mid-parent is ***half*** of additive variance.

135. Selection for combining ability is known as ***reciprocal recurrent*** selection.

136. The genetic covariance of full sib is $\frac{1}{2} V_A + 1/4 V_D$.

137. Milk yield and fat percentage are ***negatively*** correlated traits.

138. ***Variation*** is hope and despair of animal breeder.

139. Quantitative traits are generally governed by ***several*** number of genes.

5

Animal Genetics and Breeding Principles of Genetics & Population Genetics

Q.1. True and False

1.	False	Epitasis is an intra-allelic interaction.
2.	False	In small population in absence of migration, mutation and selection gene frequencies do not change over the generations.
3.	False	The component of genetic variation is V_P and V_E.
4.	True	Inversion is an example of structural aberration in chromosome.
5.	False	Heritability estimate obtained by half-sib method is more than that obtained by full sib method.
6.	True	Inheritance mediated by plasmid is an example of cytoplasmic inheritance.
7.	True	In absence of over dominance the total range of value attributed to a locus is 2a.
8.	True	The places in DNA most prone to mutation are called as hot spots.
9.	False	Population mean is not affected by gene frequency.
10.	False	Diploid (2n) chromosome number in chicken is 39.
11.	False	Meiosis takes place in somatic cells.
12.	True	In a population under H-W equilibrium the frequency of heterozygotes cannot be more than 0.5.

13.	False	Heritability of trait does not change over generations in a selection experiment.
14.	False	Sister chromatid exchange and translocation are same.
15.	True	Conversion of purines to pyrimidines is called transversion.
16.	False	In F-test, the sum of squares can never be negative values.
17.	True	Sex differentiation system used in poultry is ZZ and ZW.
18.	False	Selection cannot change the gene frequency.
19.	True	The ratio of 9:6:1 is obtained in duplicate gene with interaction.
20.	False	Creepers in fowl is example of mutation in poultry.
21.	True	Gene frequency refers to the relative abundance or relative rarity of a particular gene in a population as compared to its own allele.
22.	False	Egg production in poultry is sex linked trait.
23.	False	X-ray is not a mutagenic agent.
24.	True	Panmixia is a mating system in which each individual has an equal opportunity to mate with any individual of the opposite sex.
25.	True	If the polled animal had a horned parent, it must be heterozygous, as the horned parent transmits only the recessive allele for horn.
26.	True	Most reproductive traits have low heritability (0 to 15 percent).
27.	True	Mendel had no knowledge of physical nature of the genetic material when, in 1865 he promulgated his two laws.
28.	False	Swamp and water buffaloes have similar number of chromosomes.
29.	True	Quantitative traits are governed by polygenes.
30.	True	Genotype is the particular assemblage of genes possessed by the individual.
31.	True	The ratio between individual components to the total phenotypic variance is the intraclass correlation.

32.	False	For the law of independent assortment, Mendel used monohybrid crosses.
33.	True	Roan shorthorn cattle are heterozygous for an allelic pair.
34.	True	Haemophilia disease in man is controlled by a sex linked recessives gene.
35.	True	Aneuploid animals are characterized by incomplete genomes.
36.	False	Cockerels are heterogametic.
37.	True	Sex influenced heredity has to do with genes in autosome chromosomes.
38.	False	Genes with additive effects are not inherited from parent to offspring.
39.	True	Panmixia is the synonym for random mating.
40.	True	The concept of heritability was given by Lush.
41.	True	Repeatability is always higher than heritability.
42.	True	The x-ray induced mutations were reported by H.J.Muller.
43.	False	Baldness in human is due to sex linked genes.
44.	False	A chromosomal fragment lacking centromere is known as acrocentric.
45.	True	In hemizygous condition, only one allele of a pair is present as in sex linkage.
46.	False	In independent assortment, proportions of parental types are always more than recombinants.
47.	True	Selection is least effective against a recessive gene when it is rare in the population.
48.	True	Alfred H.Sturtevant published first chromosomal map.
49.	True	Extra chromosomal inheritance is non Mendelian inheritance.
50.	True	During the reductional division chromosomes are halved while in equational division chromatids are also halved.
51.	False	A small population takes one generation of random mating to reach equilibrium, provided there is no mutation, migration and selection.

52.	False	Inheritance of baldness in man is controlled by sex limited genes.
53.	True	Snail coiling is an example of cytoplasmic inheritance.
54.	True	Genetic properties of a population are expressible in the terms of gene frequencies and genotype frequencies.
55.	True	The structural aberrations include deficiencies, duplications, inversions and translocations.
56.	True	Oncogenes cause cancer.
57.	False	During crossing over there is exchange of chromosomal segments between sister chromatids of a chromosome.
58.	False	Milk production in cow is a sex linked trait.
59.	True	Three point crosses are used to determine the order of genes on a chromosome.
60.	True	Transformation involves the uptake of naked DNA molecules from one bacterium to another.
61.	False	In meiosis, first separation of sister chromatids takes place.
62.	True	If fitness of a genotype is one, then its selection coefficient will be zero.
63.	False	Expressivity is the proportion of individuals of given genotype that exhibits a given phenotype.
64.	True	In birds, female is heterogametic sex.
65.	True	Pleiotropy refers to the situation in which a gene influences more than one trait.
66.	True	A large random mating population takes one generation to reach equilibrium provided there is no mutation migration and selection.
67.	True	Crossing over occurs between non sisters chromatids.
68.	True	H.J.Muller reported that the X-ray induces mutation.
69.	True	In single locus two alleles linkage can be tested by test crossing the heterozygotes.
70.	True	Homologous chromosomes similar in both sexes are called autosomes.

71. False The physical basic unit of heredity is DNA.

72. True The normal DNA structure discovered by Watson and Crick in 1953 was B-DNA.

73. False In poultry males are heterogametic for sex chromosomes.

74. True Bateson coined the term "GENETICS".

75. False Preformation theory was given by Swammardam.

76. True Eugenic is betterment of mankind/human race.

77. True Genes for sex influenced traits are present on autosomes.

78. True Pangenesis theory had provided further explanation of new heritable changes leading to origin of new species.

79. False Restoration of same number of chromosomes after fertilization is the significance of mitosis.

80. False Maternal effects are common in mammals and can be ignored in planning breeding programme.

81. True In traits where test cross is not possible the individual is mated to known heterozygote to ascertain the presence of the recessive gene.

82. True The degree of resemblance between sibs is expressed as intraclass correlation, which is within group variance.

83. True After selection the total frequency is not zero because there is a proportional loss of square due to selection.

84. False The average effect of gene substitution is small when the frequency of recessive allele is high.

85. False Robert Hook discovered the cell in 1765.

86. True Chromosome number of camel is 74.

87. True Chromosome number of poultry is 78.

88. False Law of purity of gametes is universally not accepted.

89. True Ratio for complementary gene action is 9:7.

90. False In Hardy Weinberg law, gene and genotype frequencies are not same from generation to generation.

91. False Breeding value is a property of gene and not of a individual.

92. True Term heterosis was given by George H. Shull.

93. True Holandric genes are situated on Y chromosomes.

Q.2. Multiple Choice Questions :

1. In case of H-W equilibrium which of following is correct :

   a. P + 1/2H=1 **b. P +q = 1**

   c. P+1/2H=p d. P = p+Q

2. At equilibrium gene frequency (q) in case in pea of mutation is:

   a. v+u/u **b. u/u+v**

   c. u/v d. u+v/v

3. The seven characters which Mendel choses in pea were located on:

   a. Same chromosome b. Cytoplasm

   c. Different chromosomes d. All of the above

4. Holandric inheritance is:

   a. X-linked b. Autosomal

   c. Y-linked d. Cytoplasmic

5. Population mean depends upon:

   a. Gene frequency b. Gene action

   c. Both a & b d. None of the above

6. Purine bases in DNA are:

   a. A & G b. A & T

   c. C & T d. C & G

7. Degree of dominance may be expressed as:

   a. d/a b. a/d

   c. c+d/a d. a+d/d

8. The number of generations of selection required to reach the desired frequency is:

   a. t=1/qo **b. t=1/qt+1/qo**

   c. t=1q0-1/qt d. t=1/qt x 1/q

10. Heritability of a trait depends on:
    a. Gene frequency
    b. Gene action
    c. Mating system
    d. All of the above
11. Coupling and repulsion are related on:
    a. Multiple allelism
    b. Linkage
    c. Selection
    d. Epistasis
12. Blood group system in human being is an example of:
    a. Multiple allelism
    b. Linkage
    c. Selection
    d. Epistasis
13. Centimorgan is a:
    a. Unit
    b. Name of scientist
    c. Stage in meiosis
    d. Structural gene
14. Which of following is true for multiple alleles:
    a. Present on different loci
    b. Do not cross over
    c. Present on different chromosomes
    d. They are non allelic
15. Exchange of genetic material in bacteria which is mediated by phages is called as:
    a. Transduction
    b. Conjugation
    c. Transition
    d. Transformation
16. Duplicate gene interaction in epistasis have ratio of:
    a. 15:1
    b. 9:6:1
    c. 9:3:3:1
    d. 9:7
17. The number of characters in sweat pea considered by mendal in his experiment is:
    a. 16
    b. 9
    c. 7
    d. 13

18. ABO blood group in human being is the classical example of:

    a. Multiple factor
    b. Cytoplasmic inheritance
    c. Epistasis
    d. Multiple allele

19. The classical mendelian ratio in a dihybrid is:

    a. 9:3:3:1
    b. 15:1
    c. 13:3
    d. 9:7

20. Extra chromosomal inheritance is often called as:

    a. Non chromosomal inheritance
    b. Cytoplasmic inheritance
    c. Non mendalian inheritance
    d. All of the above

21. The chromosome number in mule is:

    a. 51
    b. 62
    c. 63
    d. 74

22. When one gene of a pair masks the presence and prevent the manifestation of its allele:

    a. Multiple allele
    b. Multiple factor
    c. Epistasis
    d. Complementary gene action

23. Which one of the following branches of genetics has relatively more direct importance in animal improvement:

    a. Cytogenesis and molecular genetics.
    b. Biochemical genetics and immunogenetics
    c. Population genetics and quantitative genetics
    d. Microbial genetics and developmental genetics

24. Which one of the following two species have 60 chromosome numbers:

    a. Cattle and yak
    b. Goat and sheep
    c. Cattle and goat
    d. Ass and horse

25. Which one of the following conditions is met for the Hardy Weinberg law:

    a. Large population
    b. Random mating

c. The absence of any force acting to change gene frequency

d. All of the above

26. Which one of the following condition applies to Mendel's second law:

a. Segregation of one locus does not influence segregation at another

b. Genes controlling separate traits segregate independently

c. Inheritance of characters controlled by separate gene pairs.

d. All of the above

27. Spotting pattern found in Holstein Friesian cattle is determined by a:

a. Recessive allele b. Dominant allele

c. Multiple alleles d. Co-dominant allele

28. Which one of the following mating is dihybrid cross:

a. BB x bb **b. BB DD x bb dd**

c. bb x bb d. None of the above

29. When pure bred red coat colour short horn cattle is mated to pure white's coat colour it give uniform F_1 that is:

a. Unlike either parent b. Red

c. White **d. Roan**

30. Heritability of milk yield is:

a. High **b. Medium**

c. Low d. Zero

31. F_2 ratio in dominant recessive epistasis is:

a. 12:3:1 b. 9:6:1

c. 13:3 d. 9:7

32. Four linkage groups are found in:

a. Cattle b. Buffalo

c. Poultry **d. Drosophila**

33. Mutation occurs in:

a. Somatic cells b. Reproductive cells

c. Both of the above d. None of the above

34. Multiple alleles are the genes:
    a. Having more than two forms of a gene
    b. Situated on the same locus
    c. Resulting in more than two genotypes
    d. All of the above

35. Johannsen coined the term:
    a. Genotype
    b. Gene
    c. Phenotype
    d. All of the above

36. A multiple allelic locus has 3 alleles, the possible genotypes are:
    a. 6
    b. 5
    c. 4
    d. 3

37. In dihybrid segregation analysis we deal with:
    a. Multiple locus
    b. Single locus
    c. Double locus
    d. None of the above

38. A population cannot be in H-W equilibrium if it is:
    a. Open
    b. Small
    c. Mutating
    d. None of the above

39. The effectiveness of gene exchange under migration depends upon:
    a. The number of individuals migrated
    b. Difference in gene frequencies between native and migrated population
    c. Both a & b
    d. None of the above

40. The regression coefficient between two variables is independent of :
    a. Origin
    b. Scale
    c. Both a & b
    d. Neither

41. The germ plasma theory of inheritance was proposed by:
    a. Darwin
    b. Lamark
    c. August Weismann
    d. Galton

42. The diploid chromosome number in cattle is:

a. 60 b. 50

c. 30 d. 25

43. Crossing over takes place during:

a. Metaphase–I b. Anaphase–I

c. Pachytene of prophase–I d. Prophase–II

44. Turner's syndrome is characterized by:

a. Triploidy chromosome–21

b. Trisomy of chromosome–21

c. Monosomy of sex chromosome

d. Trisomy of sex chromosome

45. Barred plumage in poultry is a:

a. Sex-limited trait. b. Sex-influenced trait

c. Sex-linked trait d. None of the above

46. Gene transcription takes place in:

a. Nucleus b. Ribosomes

c. Golgi apparatus d. Centrosomes

47. In tri-hybrid cross the number of different kinds of genotypes in F_2 are:

a. 3 **b. 27**

c. 8 d. 9

48. In case of non-linked genes:

a. Only parental combinations are produced

b. **Parental and new combinations in equal frequency**

c. Parental combinations always more than the new combinations

d. New combinations always more than the parental combinations

49. Accepting a false hypothesis is:

a. Type-I error **b. Type-II error**

c. Both of the above d. None of the above

50. In RBD experiment analysis of variance will consists of:

    a. Two-way analysis of variance

    b. Three-way analysis of variance

    c. Factorial analysis

    d. One- way analysis of variance

51. The term gene was coined by:

    a. Wilhelm Johannsen b. George Mendel

    c. Hardy-Weinberg d. Lush

52. The proportion of sex linked genes in a population is:

    a. Higher in heterogametic sex

    b. Higher in homogametic sex

    c. Equal in both sexes

    d. None of the above

53. The number of chromosomes in trisomic cattle would be equal to:

    a. 59 b. 60

    c. 61 d. 62

54. For gene mapping we need:

    a. Single cross over frequencies

    b. Double cross over frequencies

    c. Both of the above

    d. None of the above

55. Epistasis ratio of 9:7 is observed in:

    a. Recessive epistasis

    b. Duplicate recessive epistasis

    c. Dominant recessive epistasis

    d. None of the above

56. Hardy Weinberg equilibrium in a population can be achieved if it is:

    a. Random mating b. Close

    c. Large **d. All of the above**

57. A simplest type of operating system is:

a. Multiprogramming
b. Single user multi task
c. Single user single task
d. Multi user single task

58. Test of significance for small paired sample means is:

a. Chi-square test
b. T-test
c. Z-test
d. F-test

59. Sex linked alleles cannot be passed from a :

a. Woman to her daughters
b. Man to his grandsons
c. Man to his sons
d. Woman to her grand daughters

60. A 9:3:4 F_2 ratios in dihybrid cross is observed in:

a. Recessive epitasis
b. Dominant epitasis
c. Complementary gene action
d. None of the above

61. Mendel interpreted the results with pea as demonstrating:

a. Blending inheritance
b. Particulate inheritance
c. Cytoplasmic inheritance
d. None of the above

62. A ratio of X chromosomes to autosomes in a drosophila is 0.5 then it will be a:

a. Female
b. Male
c. Inter sex
d. Super male

63. How many types of gametes a genotype aaBBCCdd can produce (assuming independent assortment):

a. 4
b. 8
c. 9
d. 1

64. DNA replication takes place in which phase of cell cycle :

a. G_1 phase
b. G_2 phase
c. S phase
d. None of the above

65. Horn in sheep is a:

a. Sex linked trait
b. Sex limited traits
c. Sex influenced trait
d. None of the above

66. Which one from the following is chemical mutagen:

a. Neutrons
b. Ultraviolet rays
c. X-rays
d. Benzedine

67. Which one from the following is due to structural changes in the chromosome:

a. Polyploidy
b. Polysomic
c. Duplication
d. Monosomic

68. When one gene of a pair masks the presence and prevents the manifestation of its allele:

a. Multiple allele
b. Multiple factor
c. Epistasis
d. Complementary gene action

69. Mahogany and While I Red and White coat colour in cattle is controlled by:

a. Sex limited
b. Sex influenced
c. Sex linked
d. None of the above

70. Down's syndrome (Mangolism) results from:

a. Trisomic
b. Tetrasomic
c. Nullsomic
d. Double trisomic

71. In a large randomly mating population, in the absence of migration, mutation and selection, gene and genotypic frequencies remains constant generation after generation follows one of the following laws:

a. Law of dominance
b. Law of segregation
c. Law of independent assortment
d. Hardy-Weinberg law

72. A process by which parts of homologous chromosomes are interchanged and recombination of genes on the same chromosome is accomplished:

a. Interference
b. Coincidence
c. Crossing over
d. Linkage

73. The theory of inheritance of acquired characters was proposed by:

a. CharlesDarwin
b. Jean-Baptiste Lamarck
c. Weismann
d. Galton

74. The diploid chromosome number in buffalo is:

a. 60
b. 50
c. 30
d. 25

75. Down's syndrome is characterized by:

a. Triploidy of chromosome – 21
b. Trisomy of chromosome – 21
c. Monosomy of chromosome – 21
d. Deletion in chromosome -21

76. Red green colour blindness is a:

a. Sex limited trait
b. Sex influenced trait
c. Sex linked trait
d. None of the above

77. Gene translation takes place in:

a. Nucleus
b. Ribosomes
c. Golgi apparatus
d. Centrosomes

78. In dihybrid cross the number of different kinds of genotypes in F_2 are:

a. 3
b. 4
c. 8
d. 9

79. A chromosome is characterized by its:

a. Size
b. Position of centromere
c. Banding pattern
d. All of the above

80. F2 ratio observed in complementary gene action is:

a. 15:1
b. 9:7
c. 9:3:4
d. 12:3:1

81. A ratio of x chromosomes to autosomes in a drosophila is 1.0, then it will be a:

 a. Female b. Male

 c. Inter sex d. Super male

82. When bacterial genes are carried from a donor cell to a recipient cell by bacteriophage, then it is known as:

 a. Transformation **b. Transduction**

 c. Conjugation d. None of the above

83. Structural chromosomal aberrations include:

 a. Deletion and duplication b. Inversion

 c. Translocation **d. All of the above**

84. Which phase of cell cycle is usually the shortest period of the cycle:

 a. G_1 phase b. G_2 phase

 c. S phase **d. Mitosis**

85. Milk production in cattle is a:

 a. Sex linked trait **b. Sex limited trait**

 c. Sex influenced trait d. None of the above

86. Compound may be:

 a. Digital b. Analog

 c. Hybrid **d. All of the above**

87. 9:7 epistasis ratios are observed in:

 a. Recessive epistasis

 b. Duplicate recessive epistasis

 c. Dominant recessive epistasis

 d. None of the above

88. With same number of progeny, we have more confidence in suspected sire mated to with:

 a. Own daughter b. Known carrier

 c. Affected female d. None of the above

89. In cattle, how many chromosomes would be in nullsomic:

a. 59 b. 60

c. 61 d. 62

90. The test of significance used for qualitative trait is:

a. F-test b. Z-Test

c. Chi-square test d. None of the above

91. The covariance between full sibs is:

a. $0.5V_A+0.25V_D$ b. $0.5V_A+0.5V_D$

c. $0.25V_A+0.25V_D$ d. $0.25V_A+0.5VD$

92. XXY chromosome compliment is found in:

a. Down's syndrome b. Turner's syndrome

c. Klinefelter's syndrome d. Patau syndrome

93. The complete set of chromosomes found in the gamete of a diploid is called as:

a. Basic number b. Polyploidy

c. Genome d. Monosomic

94. In population genetics, we deal with:

a. Metric traits only

b. Population only

c. Casual components of variation

d. All of the above

95. When twins are produced, one of them being male and other female, female is sterile and male is normal. It is called as:

a. Dizygotic twins b. Identical twins

c. Free martin d. Monozygotic twins

96. Additive genetic variance of trait is 5000 $kg^2$and phenotypic standard deviation is 100kg then the heritability of trait would be:

a. 0.2 **b. 0.5**

c. 0.25 d. 0.16

97. W. Harvey had speculated that all animals arise from an egg and semen plays a role in it under :

a. Spontaneous theory **b. Epigenesis theory**

c. Germplasm theory d. Pangenesis theory

98. The cytological basis of crossing over in drosophila was demonstrated by:

a. B. Meclintok **b. Curt Stern**

c. M.B. Creighkton d. None of the above

99. Bateson and Punnett discovered the presence of :

a. Lethal genes b. Crossing over

c. Linkage d. Multiple genes

100. Which of the following is not an example of cytoplasmic inheritance:

a. Coiling snails **b. Colour blindness in dogs**

c. Eye colour in beach hopper d. Milk factor in mice

101. Hardy-Weinberg Law does not operate in absence of :

a. Large population b. Selection

c. Migration d. Mutation

102. Covariance of offspring and one parent is :

a. ¼ V_A **b. ½ V_A**

c. ½ V_p d. None of the above

103. During meiosis crossing over observed in:

a. Leptotene b. Zygotene

c. Pachytene d. Diplodtene

104. Cytoplasmic inheritance is due to:

a. Mitochondria b. Ribosome

c. Golgi body d. None of the above

105. ZZ-ZW sex determination occurs in:

a. Poultry b. Moth

c. Human d. None of the above

106. Father of genetics is:

A. T. H. Morgan **b. G. J. Mendel**

c. H.J.Muller d. G.H. Shull

107. Chromosome number of goat is:

a. 50 b. 58

c. 60 d. 68

108. Which blood group system in human being is an example of multiple alleles:

a. ABO b. ACD

c. Rh d. ZZ

109. The genes located on X-chromosome are called as:

a. Sex linked b. Sex limited

c. Sex influenced d. Holandric

110. An exception to Mendel's law is:

a. Independent assortment b. Dominance

c. Segregation **d. Linkage**

111. Haemophilia in man is controlled by:

a. Sex-influenced gene **b. Sex-linked gene**

c. Sex-limited gene d. Holandric gene

112. If a plant heterozygous for tallness is selfed, the F2 generation is both tall:

a. Dominance **b. Segregation**

c. Independent assortment d. Incomplete dominance

113. The genetic constitution of an organism is known as:

a. Genetic code **b. Genotype**

c. Phenotype d. Gene pool

114. Most important force for changing gene frequency in a population is:

a. Chance b. Mutation

c. Selection **d. Migration**

Q.3. Fill in the Blanks

1. In poultry heterogametic sex is ***female.***
2. The total variance Vp can be partitioned into $V_G + V_E$.
3. The gene balance theory is related to ***sex determination.***
4. Coat colour in rabbit is an example of ***multiple allele.***
5. Change in gene frequency Dq due to migration is ***m(qm-qo).***
6. In paternal half sib method the correlation among sib is **¼.**
7. In dihybrid cross ***two*** pair(s) of genes are involved.
8. The average of gene substitution ***a = a1-a2.***
9. The h^2 in narrow sense is V_A/V_P
10. The chromosome in which centromere is located in the middle is called as ***metacentric.***
11. Barr bodies are visible in ***female*** mammals.
12. Increase in total chromosomal set beyond diploid is called ***polyploidy.***
13. Presence of more than two alleles on same locus is called ***multiple alleles.***
14. Inheritance of comb shape in poultry is an example of ***epistasis.***
15. In case of no dominance change in gene frequency Dq due tone generation of selection is ***-1/2sq (1-q)/1-sq.***
16. P(AB)=P(A). P(B/A)=P (B). P(A/B) is the theorem of ***compound probability.***
17. The inheritance of barred plumage in poultry is a classical example of ***sex linkage*** inheritance.
18. The honey bee (queen, workers and drone) is a classical example of ***parthenogenesis.***
19. ***Oncogenes*** cause cancer in human being.
20. Cat cry syndrome in human being is associated with ***deletion*** in chromosomes.
21. Inheritance of baldness in man is controlled by ***sex limited*** genes
22. The ratio of 15:1 is obtained in the ***duplicate dominant*** epistasis.

23. In chicken, male possesses two X-chromosome whereas female possesses only ***one.***

24. ***Population genetics*** is the study of mendalian genetics in population of animals or plants.

25. ***G.H Hardy and W. Weinberg*** were the basic founders of population genetics.

26. Changes in the genetic information carried by a cell are called ***mutation.***

27. ***Pleiotropy*** is defined as a single allele influencing more than one distinct trait.

28. When gene and genotype frequencies remain constant in a population is said to be ***equilibrium.***

29. ***Gene frequency*** is the proportion of the total number of genes represented by a particular allele.

30. A line graph of class frequency plotted against class mark is a ***frequency polygon.***

31. Dispersive changes in gene frequency occur in ***small*** population.

32. Selection for a recessive gene is ***difficult*** in comparison to selection for a dominant gene.

33. Extra parts of chromosomes are called ***duplication.***

34. ***Translocation*** is the phenomenon of transfer of a section of one chromosome to a non homologous chromosome.

35. Regression of breeding value on phenotypic value is ***heritability.***

36. The shortest of the mitotic phases is the ***anaphase.***

37. A trait is inherited in a crisscross manner is ***sex linked*** inheritance.

38. ***Heritability*** is the ratio of additive genetic variance to total phenotypic variance.

39. The three systematic processes that can change the gene frequency are ***mutation, migration and selection.***

40. The genotype frequency ranges from ***0 to 1.***

41. If the frequency of A_1 and A_2 alleles in a population under H.W. equilibrium are 0.7 and 0.3, respectively, then the frequency of A_1A_1, A_1A_2 and A_2, A_2 genotypes shall be ***0.49, 0.42 and 0.09,*** respectively.

42. The phenomenon is which a gene pair is suppressed by another gene pair is called ***epistasis.***

43. Crossing over is absent in ***male*** drosophila.

44. Red, green colour blindness in man is a ***sex linked*** trait.

45. The part of the chromosome which is genetically active and less coiled is called ***euchromatin.***

46. Number of linkage group corresponds with ***haploid*** chromosome number of that species.

47. Structural chromosomal abnormality occurs due to ***translocation.***

48. The diploid number of chromosomes in a sheep is ***54.***

49. Heterozygous superiority is due to ***overdomiance.***

50. Presence of horn in some breeds of sheep is ***sex influenced.***

51. In single locus with two alleles if AA and Aa are 64 percent, then frequency of ***A*** gene will be ***0.4.***

52. Breeding value is ***half*** of the transmitting ability.

53. The proportion of recessive homozygous (aa) in a population is 64 per cent, then the frequency of *A* gene will be ***0.2*** in a single locus two alleles case.

54. Heritability (narrow sense) is a ratio of ***additive genetic variance and phenotypic variance.***

55. ABO blood group system in man is an example of ***multiple alleles.***

56. Different types of gametes produced by a drosophila male when only one locus on each chromosome is heterozygous ***16.***

57. If an allele A is fixed in the population then its gene frequency will be ***1.0.***

58. Intra allelic interaction is known as ***dominance.***

59. One map unit = ***1.0 % recombination frequency.***

60. ***Mutation*** is a sudden heritable change in the structure of the genetic material.

61. The coat colour in rabbit is a classical example of ***multiple allele.***

62. Structural aberration of chromosome includes ***deletion, inversion, duplication and translocation.***
63. Other than chromosomal, inheritance is called as ***cytoplasmic inheritance.***
64. The alternative state at the same locus is known as ***multiple*** alleles.
65. Duplicate gene with interaction in epistasis have phenotypic ratio of ***9:6:1***
66. Creeper fowl is example of ***lethal gene.***
67. If the frequencies of A1 and A2 alleles in a population under H.W equilibrium are ***0.6 and 0.4*** the frequency of A_1A_1, A_1A_2 and A_2A_2 genotypes shall be 0.36, 0.48 and 0.16 respectively.
68. The phenomenon in which one gene affects several traits is called ***pleiotropism.***
69. The phenotypic variance is equal to genotypic variance plus ***environmental variance.***
70. Barred plumage in poultry is a ***sex linked*** trait.
71. Mendel's principle in which linkage is violated ***independent assortment.***
72. Sudden heritable change in the genetic material is known as ***mutation.***
73. The heritability of a trait ranges from ***0 to1.***
74. In mammals ***sex linked recessive*** traits are observed more frequently in males than females.
75. The diploid chromosome number in water buffalo is ***50.***
76. In a single locus two allele case the frequency of a will be ***0.5*** if AA and Aa genotypes are 75%.
77. Additive genetic variance is ***¼*** of sire variance.
78. Example of sex influenced trait in sheep is ***presence of horn.***
79. Number of linkage groups of a species corresponds with ***haploid*** chromosome member.
80. Crossing over takes place in ***pachytene*** stage of prophase–I.
81. ***A, B, and O*** blood groups system in human beings is an example of multiple allele.

82. Regression of offspring on mid-parent value is equal to ***heritability.***

83. A coiled filament throughout the length of a chromosome is known as ***chromonemata.***

84. The effect of sex hormones in sex limited traits is whether the trait will be ***expressed or not.***

85. Inheritance of ***measurable*** traits that depends on the cumulative action of many ***genes*** is the quantitative inheritance.

86. The breeding value of an individual is equal to the ***sum*** of average of ***genes*** it carries.

87. The difference between the ***covariance*** of the full sibs and half sibs provides a way of estimating the dominance deviation.

88. The difference between the frequencies in sex linked genes is half the difference between the frequencies in the ***previous*** generation but in the ***opposite*** direction.

89. Pairing of homologous chromosome takes place in ***zygotene*** stage of prophase I of meiosis.

90. Terms linkage and crossing over proposed by ***Thomas Hunt Morgan.***

91. Sum of gene frequency is always equal to ***1.***

92. Range of gene frequency is ***0 to 1.***

93. Cause of variation in population is mainly due to genetic and ***environmental factors.***

94. If a gene occurs in more than two alternative forms or alleles, it is known to exhibit ***multiple allelism.***

95. The position or place on a chromosome occupied by a particular gene or one of its alleles is known as ***locus.***

96. The term genetics was coined by ***William Bateson*** in 1909.

97. The genotypic ratio of a monohybrid cross will be ***1:2:1.***

98. Gregor Mendel is called ***father of genetics.***

99. F_2 ratio in a dihybrid cross will be ***9:3:3:1.***

100. Criss-cross inheritance is observed in ***sex linked*** heredity.

101. The ratio of additive genetic variance to ***total phenotypic variance*** is referred as h^2.

102. Epistasis is ***inter allelic/non-allelic.***

103. The external or outward expression is called as ***phenotype.***

104. When a gene marks the expression of its own allele, phenomena is called ***dominance.***

6

Animal Nutrition (PART-I) Principles of Animal Nutrition Feed & Feed Technology

Q.1. Write "True" or "False" against each Statement

1. False "Thumps" is commonly seen in calves.
2. False Animal calorimeter was developed by Kellner.
3. False Feeding of large quantity of wheat bran may lead to phosphorus deficiency.
4. False Osteoporosis is caused due to deficiency of iron.
5. True Zinc deficiency leads to "parakeratosis" in pigs.
6. False Enamel of the teeth contains 10% moisture.
7. True Per mole of butyric acid after complete metabolism produces 25 moles of ATP.
8. True Thiamine is a sulphur containing vitamin.
9. False Measurement of ME accounts only fecal loss.
10. False NE value of feed for maintenance and fattening are same.
11. False R.Q. value of 0.7 is an indicative of CHO metabolism in the body.
12. False Starch equivalent is a measure of metabolizable energy.
13. False In EAAI method, only most deficient essential amino acid is considered.
14. False Crops rich in soluble carbohydrate are not suitable for silage making.

15.	False	Chitin is the principle component of the exoskeleton of bacteria.
16.	True	Main source of bicarbonate phosphate buffer in ruminants is saliva.
17.	False	Molasses is most suitable carbohydrate for protein synthesis.
18.	False	The ability of liver and other tissues to store sugar as glycogen is unlimited.
19.	True	Utilization of urea is much less in high protein rations, particularly where soluble proteins are present.
20.	False	Lignin is not resistant to chemical degradation.
21.	True	Pantothenic acid is a constituent of coenzyme A.
22.	True	Deamination occurs extensively in liver.
23.	True	Linoleic acid is essential at tissue level.
24.	False	Excessive intake of essential fatty acids does not lead to increased Vit. E requirement.
25.	True	Roughages are low in crude protein content.
26.	True	Mixed glucans are present in the cell wall.
27.	True	Sufficient dry matter is lost due to white rot fungi treatment of wheat straw.
28.	False	Urea treatment of straw is better than the urea (ammonition) ensiling.
29.	False	Biological value of protein is not a better quality measure.
30.	False	Green fodder to be ensiled should have 10-20 percent water.
31.	True	Heat of combustion of carbohydrate is 4.15 Kcal/g of mixed diet.
32.	False	All the alkaloids have poisonous property.
33.	False	Nitrates as such are toxic to animals.
34.	False	Only few amino acids occurring naturally in proteins are of the a type.
35.	False	Carotenes are absorbed from the gut as efficiently as Vit. A.
36.	True	Mature hay and straw are rich in lignin.

37.	True	Concentrates are poor source of crude fibre.
38.	True	Crystalline cellulose is better degraded than amorphous cellulose.
39.	True	White rot fungi degrades carbohydrate and lignin both.
40.	True	Alkali treatment is no more economic and effective as compared to other chemicals for the treatment of poor quality roughages.
41.	True	Sulphuric and hydrochloric acids are used in AIV silage making.
42.	True	The moisture content of good quality hay should not exceed 20 percent.
43.	False	The cell wall of plants and cell membrane of animals are chiefly cellulose.
44.	True	Oxidation of one gram fat yields more than one gram metabolic water.
45.	False	Lignin is a carbohydrate.
46.	True	Amino acids are amphoteric.
47.	False	Feed additives are nutrients and can be considered as dietary essential.
48.	False	Plants get their energy from soil.
49.	True	Volatile fatty acids are the major source of energy in ruminants.
50.	True	Biological measure reflects the content of limiting amino acids in protein.
51.	True	Pellated feeds are usually less dusty and more palatable.
52.	True	R.Q. value below 0.7 is observed in fasting animals.
53.	False	Cereal grains are usually higher in calcium than phosphorus.
54.	True	Feeding of poor quality roughages result in large proportion of energy lost as methane.
55.	False	Bomb calorimeter is also used for the measurement of heat increments in ruminants.
56.	True	White rot fungi is commonly used for improving the nutritive value of crop residues.

57. True — *Daily water requirement of adult hens is double the quantity of DM consumed.*

58. False — *Acetic acid is a glucogenic acid.*

59. True — *Oxidation of 1gm glucose yield 0.6gm metabolic water.*

60. False — *Oligosaccharides contain more than 10 sugar units.*

61. True — *Starch is the only polysaccharide which can be utilized by monogastric animals.*

62. True — *The major role of Vitamin D is in the calcium and phosphorus metabolism.*

63. True — *Carbohydrates make up about 75 percent of the dry matter of the plants.*

64. False — *Fat is not necessary in a ruminant diet.*

65. True — *Deficiency of minerals and vitamins may interfere with energy utilization.*

66. False — *Losses of energy in the urine is inversely proportional to the protein content of the feed.*

67. True — *The NE values for maintenance and lactation are higher than for growth.*

68. False — *Metabolizable energy will be utilized more efficiently for maintenance in ruminants than in non-gastric animals.*

69. False — *Heat production in an animal is not related to body size.*

70. True — *A ratio of energy to protein exerts an influence on feed intake and feed efficiency.*

71. False — *Steamed bone meal is a good source of protein.*

72. False — *Bile is synthesized in the gall bladder and function in fat metabolism.*

73. False — *Erepsin is an enzyme secreted from the wall of duodenum.*

74. True — *Vitamin D helps in the synthesis of specific messenger RNA.*

75. True — *Bran and oil cakes are rich source of magnesium.*

76. True — *Tyrosine is an a-amino b-hydroxyl phenyl propoionic-acid.*

77. False — *The process of amino acid-keto acid conversion is termed* transamination.

78.	True	Megacalory and thern are the same.
79.	True	The biological value of meat meal is lower than that of fish meal.
80.	False	Carotenoids substance are added to feed to improve growth of broiler and pullets.
81.	True	Chunies are self balance ration for live-stock.
82.	True	L-plantarum and enterobacter spp. are known to reduce nitrate to nitrite in the silage.
83.	True	Tank age is an ideal supplement for swine.
84.	False	Linseed is rich in linoleic acid.
85.	False	The term biological value was first applied to protein by William Prout.
86.	False	Million's test is performed to test the presence of tryptophan.
87.	False	Protein is having on average about 6.25 % nitrogen.
88.	True	Leguminous fodder is unfit for silage making.
89.	False	Cereal grains are rich in calcium and phytate.
90.	False	Glycogen is a common component of many feed.
91.	True	The energy value of feed is expressed in term of TDN.
92.	False	The name of berseem is Indian clover.
93.	False	*Cyonopsis tetragonoloba* is important drought resistant legume fodder for Rabi crop.
94.	True	*Stylosanthes gracilis* is a vigorous summer growing perennial grass for range pasture.
95.	False	Oxygen gas is essential for the production of good silage.
96.	True	Fodder harvested at full bloom stage is more suitable for hay making.
97.	False	PER values are the same as GPV value for protein and ME.
98.	True	ARC feeding standard are based on DCP, AP, DE and ME.
99.	False	Thayer's was the first American scientist who developed feeding standard.
100.	False	FU standard was used for energy by German scientist.

101. True — Fodder used for making silage is having 35 percent moisture.

102. True — The nutritive value of paddy straw crude protein is zero for livestock.

103. False — The end products of carbohydrate digestion in ruminants are glucose, methane and carbon dioxide.

104. True — As the animal body matures, its fat content increases and water contents decreases.

105. False — In plants the structural component is cellulose and the reserve material is protein.

106. False — All unsaturated fatty acids are essential fatty acids.

107. False — In birds the principal end product of nitrogen metabolism is urea.

108. True — α-tocopherol is a natural biological antioxidant.

109. False — In poultry crushing and grinding of feed takes place in the crop.

110. True — Propionic acid is glucogenic in nature.

111. True — RDP stands for rumen degradable protein.

112. True — The nutritive value of forage decreases with the maturity.

113. True — Legume roughages are in general good source of protein and calcium.

114. True — Heat of nutrient metabolism is a component of heat increment.

115. True — Protein efficiency ratio is defined as the weight gain per unit weight of protein eaten.

116. False — The metabolisable energy values for maintenance and lactation are lower than for growth.

117. False — Good quality silage is prepared only from leguminous fodders.

118. False — Feed material can be stored safely when moisture content is more than 15 percent.

119. True — Starch is the most important storage form of carbohydrate in the plant kingdom.

120. False — Folacin or folic acid is not readily destroyed by heat.

121. True — Vitamin B_{12} is found almost exclusively in foods/feeds of animal origin.

122. False — The biological activity of synthetic vitamin is not the same as that of the naturally occurring vitamin.

123. True — When consumed in excess, fat soluble vitamins tend to store in the body whereas water soluble vitamins get excreted in the urine.

124. False — Vitamin-A has been found only in materials of plant origin.

125. True — A slight deficiency of riboflavin in chick's results in *curled toe* paralysis.

126. True — Deficiency of pantothenic acid in pigs leads to a characteristic gait of *goose stepping.*

127. True — The principle behind TDN system of expressing feed energy is the same as proposed by Hanneberg and Stohmann.

128. True — The metabolic fecal nitrogen is expressed on the basis of per unit dry matter consumed.

129. True — The biological values of feedstuffs primarily depend on their amino acid content and also the protein level in the test diet.

130. True — Nitrogen excretion via the urine is known by endogenous urinary nitrogen on a nitrogen free diet.

131. False — The biological value of whole egg proteins is inferior to that of the whole milk.

132. False — Digestible energy is the gross energy of the undigested portion of the feedstuff.

133. False — One kilocalorie represents the amount of heat needed to raise the temperature of one gram water by 1^0C.

134. False — Bomb calorimeter is the device used to measure protein quality of feeds.

135. True — Water is an essential nutrient.

136. True — Absorption of carbohydrates is by active transport as well as passive diffusion.

137. True — Monosaccharides are the end products of carbohydrate metabolism.

138. False Linoleic acid is an essential amino acid.

139. False Elastins are present in skin, tendons and connective tissue.

140. True Parturient paresis is caused by calcium deficiency.

141. False Iron is also termed as anti-pernicious anaemia factor.

142. False Feed additives are nutritive substances, which are added to basal feed to improve its utilization.

143. True Cow pea and berseem are leguminous fodder crops.

144. False Lime stone powder is a good source of phosphorus.

145. False Armsby feeding standard is based on starch equivalent.

146. False Energy content of feeds can be estimated in colorimeter

147. False Haylages have 60-65% moisture.

148. True Groundnut oil cakes are highly susceptible to aflatoxin contamination.

149. True The *Brassica* species usually contain goitrous anti-nutritional factors.

150. False The efficiency of utilization of metabolizable energy for lactation is greater than for maintenance.

151. True Essential fatty acid having C-18 chain length is linolenic acid.

152. False Sulfur containing amino acid having SH bonded is cystein.

153. True Vitamin helps in carboxylation of pyruvic acid is biotin.

154. False Biological cycle generating pentose sugars is cori cycle.

155. False Natural occurring dietary anti oxidant is BHT.

156. False Pepsin is an endoenzyme.

157. False Propionic acid is a ketogenic volatile fatty acid.

158. True Chlorophyll is a green pigment and non nutrient in nature extracted out with fat solvent.

159. False Prucic acid is a cynogenic glucoside present in mature green fodder.

160. False SE value of feed is first proposed by a scientist Armsby.

161. True EE gives 2.52 times more energy than the carbohydrate.

162. False Lignin is mostly associated with the carbohydrate and therefore categorized under carbohydrate.

163. True Ash is a natural feed indicator.

164. False Green coloured silage is due to presence of a pigment called as xanthophyll.

165. False Pelleting of feed reduces its nutritional value and increases the density of feed.

166. False Dimetridiazole is a choice of chemical agent used for partitioning of fiber in the diet.

167. True The term probiotics was coined by Parker in 1974.

168. False P.J.Van Soest (1960) estimates the proximate analysis of feed stuffs.

169. True Enamel of teeth is the hardest tissue of body.

170. True A net 17 moles of ATP is produced per mole of propionic acid metabolism.

171. False Urea (a NPN compound) is least degradable in rumen than any other protein sources like cakes etc.

172. True Grams of iodine absorbed by the 100g fat is called inodine number.

173. True Grass staggers in animals is due to magnesium deficiency.

174. True One international unit (I.U.) of vitamin D is defined as the activity of 0.025 ìg of crystalline vitamin D3.

175. True Chaffing of green forage increase the surface area for enzymatic digestion in rumen.

176. False Heat increment from feeding of roughages is less than from feeding of concentrates.

177. True Determination of TDN does not require a digestion trial but chemical analysis of feeds and faeces is required.

178. True Bound gossypol is less toxic than free gossypol.

179. True Feed richer in protein have narrow nutritive ratio.

180. False Crops with thick stem are not used for silage making.

181. True Selective feeding of a particular feed ingredient is minimized by pelleting of feed ingredients.

182. False — The feed material can be stored safely when its moisture content is less than 18 percent.

183. False — Non-ruminants can easily digest cellulosic carbohydrates in their diet.

184. False — Animals can synthesize essential amino acids in their body.

185. True — Water is the universal solvent essential for life.

186. True — The term crude protein does not distinguish between true protein and non protein nitrogen.

187. False — The term ether extract denotes true fats and oils only.

188. True — The amylopectin molecule is much larger to that of amylase molecule.

189. True — Glycogen, the storage form of carbohydrate in animals is often referred to as animal starch.

190. True — Waxes are simple lipids of no nutritive value to the animal.

191. True — Chemical composition of any feedstuff indicates its potential value but not the actual nutritive value.

192. True — Digestibility is defined as that portion of a feed or the nutrient not recovered in faeces.

193. True — Moisture content in the crop prior to hay making has an important bearing on the nutritive quality of hay.

194. True — Proper alkali treatment of cereal straws results in notable improvement of its digestibility.

195. True — The Atwater's physiological fuel values are not applicable to ruminants because the digestibility of nutrients is lower to the figures for human beings.

196. True — The term true protein is used to denote the proteinic material only.

197. True — Dietary protein not degraded in the rumen by microbial enzymes is referred to as rumen undergradable protein.

198. True — In ruminants, the significance of protein quality varies with production status for all of the essential amino acids synthesized.

199. False — Milk and green leafy crops are very poor source of calcium.

200. True Methionine is an essential amino acid in the diet of animals.

201. False Propionate is not a glucogenic acid.

202. False Urea formation takes place in kidney.

203. True Glycogen is a branched polysaccharide.

204. False Clubbed down occurs due to the deficiency of thiamine.

205. False Goiter is caused due to the deficiency of chlorine.

206. False Dry matter content of plant is mainly carbohydrates.

207. True Hay making inhibits the action of plant and microbial enzymes.

208. True Copper sulphate may be used as growth stimulator.

209. True Physical treatment of straw improves its nutrient intake and utilization.

210. True Biological value of animal protein is better than plant protein.

211. True Expression of energy in terms of ME is better than TDN.

212. False PER is the weight gain per unit weight of dry matter eaten.

213. False NPN compounds should not be added in ruminant diet.

Q.2. Multiple Choices

1. "Goose stepping" gait in pigs is due to deficiency of:

   a. Niacin b. Biotin

   c. Pantothenic acid c. Choline

2. "Crazy chick disease" is related to deficiency of:

   a. Folic acid b. Vitamin C

   c. Vitamin E d. Thiamin

3. Is referred as "Lipotropic factor":

   a. Choline b. Biotine

   c. Thiamine d. Pyridoxine

4. Curled toe paralysis in birds is due to deficiency of:

   a. Riboflavin b. Thiamine

   c. Pyridoxine d. Choline

5. "Mottling of teeth" is related with the toxicity of:

   a. Calcium **b. Fluorine**

   c. Selenium d. Sodium

6. "Blind staggers is due to toxicity of:

   a. Fluorine **b. Selenium**

   c. Molybdenum d. Calcium

7. Stringy wool" is related with the deficiency of:

   a. Fluorine b. Cobalt

   c. Copper d. Selenium

8. "Falling disease" is a chronic deficiency of:

   a. Fluorine b. Cobalt

   c. Copper d. Selenium

9. Moisture percent in good quality silage must be:

   a. 30-40% b. 40-50%

   c. 50-60% **d. 60-70%**

10. It is not a physical treatment:

    a. Grinding b. Toasting

    c. Ammoniation d. Soaking

11. The good quality silage should have pH between:

    a. 2-3 b. 3-4

    c. 4-5 d. 5-6

12. Digestibility of bacterial protein is:

    a. 80 percent **b. 74 percent**

    c. 65 percent d. 55 percent

13. The precipitate of P is in the colour of:

    a. Red b. Pink

    c. White **d. Yellow**

14. The nitrogen balance index is a measure of:

    a. BV b. PER

    c. Feed conversion efficiency d. Calorie protein ratio

15. One of the following is not a toxicant:

    a. Oxalate b. Phytate

    c. Cryptoxanthine d. Tannin

16. Most of the amino acids are absorbed from:

    a. Caecum b. Colon

    c. Rectum **d. Small intestine**

17. The crop for hay making should be harvested at the following stage:

    a. Flowering **b. Pre-flowering**

    c. Maturity d. None above

18. The average molar percentage of acetic acid produced in sheep has been reported as:

    a. 65 b. 55

    c. 75 d. 45

19. Energy requirement by the body for the production of one mole of protein is:

    a. 90.5 KJ b. 60.5 KJ

    c. 50.5 KJ **d. 83.5 KJ**

20. The optimum microbial growth takes place when concentration of ammonia nitrogen per litre of rumen liquor is

    a. 150-250 mg b. 100-200 mg

    c. 80-150 mg d. 50-100 mg

21. Oil seeds are rich sources of:

    a. Oleic acid **b. Linoleic acid**

    c. Arachidonic acid d. Butyric acid

22. The number of carbon atoms in the side chain of sterols varies from:

    a. 8 to 10 b. 15 to 20

    c. 10 to 20 d. 25 to 30

23. Complete oxidation of butyric acid to carbon dioxide and water yields:

a.	37 moles of ATP	**b.**	**25 moles of ATP**
c.	17 moles of ATP	d.	07 moles of ATP

24. Term sugar is generally restricted to those carbohydrates containing less than following number of monosaccharides:

a.	**10**	b.	20
c.	30	d.	40

25. The water content of wheat straw is about:

a.	**10 percent**	b.	15 percent
c.	20 percent	d.	25 percent

26. Crude protein content of paddy straw is about:

a.	4 percent	**b.**	**3 percent**
c.	5 percent	d.	6 percent

27. Best expression of energy requirement in ruminants is:

a.	**NE**	b.	ME
c.	DE	d.	TDN

28. Calcium content of the bone meal is (%):

a.	**25**	b.	35
c.	45	d.	15

29. Best measure of protein quality is:

a.	DCP	b.	PER
c.	**BV**	d.	PRV

30. In preparing the AIV silage pH is brought below:

a.	6	b.	5
c.	**4**	d.	3

31. Plant cell wall is made of:

a.	Pectin	b.	Tannin
c.	**Cellulose**	d.	Protein

32. One of the antinutritional materials present in forage is:

a. Calcium **b. Tannin**

c. Cellulose d. Carotene

33. Starch is most abundant in seeds, which may contain upto:

a. 25 Percent b. 50 Percent

c. 70 Percent d. 85 Percent

34. Cellulose molecule contain β-D glucose between:

a. 1000 to 1200 b. 1300 to 1400

c. 1400 to 1500 **d. 1600 to 2700**

35. Total ATP production from oxidation of one mole of glucose is:

a. 20 b. 25

c. 38 d. 48

36. For the production of each mole of protein, the energy requirement by the body is:

a. 83.5 KJ b. 60.5 KJ

c. 50.5 KJ d. 90.5 KJ

37. Oxidation of each mole of pyruvate yields:

a. 10 moles of ATP b. 12 moles of ATP

c. 17 moles of ATP d. 20 moles of ATP

38. Osteomalacia is caused due to the deficiency of:

a. Zinc **b. Calcium**

c. Vit. A d. Copper

39. The quantity of ammonia nitrogen in rumen liquor, required for the optimum microbial growth varies from:

a. 50-100 mg/L **b. 80-150 mg/L**

c. 100-200 mg/L d. 150-250 mg/L

40. Heat of combustion of carbohydrate as per Atwater and Bryant is:

a. 4.15 Kcal/gm of mixed diet b. 5.15 Kcal/gm of mixed diet

c. 6.15 Kcal/gm of mixed diet d. 3.15 Kcal/gm of mixed diet

41. The crude protein content of wheat straw is:

a. 3.25 percent b. 4.25 percent
c. 5.35 percent d. 6.25 percent

42. The crude protein of feed is estimated by multiplying the nitrogen percentage figure by:

a. 6.25 b. 7.25
c. 5.25 d. 8.25

43. Steamed bone meal contains one of the following percentage of calcium:

a. 25 % b. 35 %
c. 45 % d. 15 %

44. The normal quantity of gross energy intake lost through the methane production is:

a. 8 % b. 10 %
c. 12 % d. 6 %

45. The digestible energy provided by one gram of TDN is:

a. 3.4 K Cal b. 5.4 K Cal
c. 4.4 K Cal d. 6.4 K Cal

46. In AIV silage making, the mixture of acids is added to bring the pH below:

a. 3.0 b. 5.0
c. 4.0 d. 6.0

47. Crude fibre content of mustard cake is:

a. 8 percent b. 10 percent
c. 12 percent d. 13 percent

48. Richest source of vit. A is:

a. Wheat straw b. Ground nut cake
c. Green berseem **d. Fish liver oil**

49. Which of the following contains highest amount of thiamine:

a. Cereals b. Roughages
c. Oil cakes d. None of the above

50. Parturient paresis in dairy cows is due to:

    a. Hypocalcemia b. Hypoglycemia

    c. Hypomagnesemia d. None of the above

51. Muscular distrophy in sheep and cattle may be prevented by administering the vitamin:

    a. Vitamin A b. Vitamin C

    c. Vitamin B **d. Vitamin E**

52. Rumen protozoa derive their nitrogen from:

    a. Ammonia b. Amides

    c. Bacteria d. All of the above

53. The most important ammonia producing bacteria present in the rumen of cattle is:

    a. *Selanomonas ruminantium*

    b. *Bacteroides ruminicola*

    c. *Ruminococcus albus*

    d. *Ruminococcus flavefaciens*

54. Raw soybeans contain an antinutritional factor:

    a. Pepsin inhibitor b. Enterokinase inhibitor

    c. Trypsin inhibitor d. Amylase inhibitor

55. The equation E2.41x+9.80 for calculation of methane production in sheep was developed by:

    a. Forbes *et al* b. Webster *et al*

    c. Blaxter *et al* **d. Swift *et al***

56. Heat production of an animal can be measured by :

    a. Respiration apparatus

    b. Bomb calorimeter

    c. Respiration calorimeter

    d. Atomic absorption spectrophotometer

57. In TDN calculation, digestible ether extract in multiplied by a factor:

    a. 6.25 b. 5.65

    c. 2.25 d. 3.73

58. The term heat increment (HI) of feeding in ruminants coined by:

    a. Rubner b. Kellner

    c. Armsby d. Blaxter

59. R.Q.value more than one may be observed when:

    a. Fat is converted to carbohydrate

    b. Carbohydrate is converted to fat

    c. Carbohydrate is converted to protein

    d. Protein is converted to fat

60. Of all roughage ration, the dominant VFA in rumen is:

    a. Propionic acid b. Butyric acid

    c. Formic acid **d. Acetic acid**

61. Which of the following is used as protein supplement for feeding to livestock:

    a. Cereals b. Roughages

    c. Oil seed cakes d. Bone meal

62. Molasses is mainly used in animals feeding as:

    a. Carrier for urea impregnation

    b. Binder for pellating of feeds

    c. Sweetner for unpalatable feeds

    d. All of the above

63. Crude protein is calculated from the nitrogen by multiplying with the:

    a. 2.25 b. 5.65

    c. 3.75 **d. 6.25**

64. Selenium is associated with:

    a. Vitamin A b. Vitamin C

    c. Vitamin E d. Vitamin K

65. Net gain of ATP from 1 ml of acetic acid metabolized:

a. 10 ATPS b. 20 ATPS

c. 25 ATPS d. 17 ATPS

66. Slipped tendon in poultry is due to deficiency syndrome of:

a. Zinc b. Copper

c. Manganese d. Magnesium

67. Ribose is a:

a. 3-carbon sugar **b. 5-carbon sugar**

c. 6 carbon sugar d. 8-carbon sugar

68. Antipernicious anemia vitamin is:

a. Vitamin B_{12} b. Vitamin B_1

c. Vitamin B_2 d. Vitamin B_6

69. Polyneuritis in birds may be due to deficiency of:

a. Vitamin A b. Vitamin D

c. Vitamin B_{12} **d. Vitamin B_1**

70. Peptide linkage is formed between:

a. Two mono saccharides

b. One amino acid and one fatty acid

c. Two amino acids

d. Two fatty acids

71. A feed stuff called roughage contains CF on IM basis more than:

a. 10 percent b. 15 per cent

c. 18 per cent d. 22 per cent

72. The chemical used in Van Soest method of partitioning of carbohydrates:

a. CTAB b. EDTA

c. RHC d. None of the above

73. Suitable crops for making good silage:

a. Maize/sorghum/oat

b. Barseem/lucerne/cowpea

c. Roots crops/doob grass/tree leaves

d. All of the above

74. The lactic acid content of silage DM is:

a. 4-6 % **b. 8-12 %**

c. 16-20 % d. Above 30 %

75. Factor used for calculation of ME from DE in ruminants:

a. 0.52 b. 0.62

c. 0.72 **d. 0.82**

76. Percent of GE intake is lost in urine in cattle:

a. 2-3 **b. 4-5**

c. 6-8 d. 10-12

77. Crude protein content of fish meal is about:

a. 30 % b. 10 %

c. 60 % d. 90 %

78. The efficiency of conversion of ME to milk is:

a. 40-50 % b. 20-30 %

c. 60-70 % d. 80-90 %

79. On hydrolysis heparin yields:

a. Sulphuric acid b. Hyaluronic acid

c. Citric acid d. Nitric acid

80. Trehalose sugar is found in:

a. Fungi b. Soyabean meal

c. Barley d. Ground nut cake

81. Cholesterol is a:

a. Phytosterol b. Mycosterol

c. Zoosterol d. Lignosterol

82. Pepsinogen is a protein digesting enzyme secreted by the:

a.	**Gastric gland**	b.	Pancrease
c.	Intestinal wall	d.	Salivary gland

83. Sunhemp leaves contain:

a.	32 percent CP	**b.**	**20 percent CP**
c.	10 percent CP	d.	5 percent CP

84. Protozoa synthesize their amino acid in the rumen from:

a.	Food nutrient	**b.**	**Bacteria**
c.	Ammonia	d.	Amino acid

85. Aflatoxin is produced by:

a.	Bacteria	**b.**	**Fungi**
c.	Mould	d.	Algae

86. The addition of substances which encourage the growth of the desirable micro organism of gastro intestinal tract is known as:

a.	Antibiotic	b.	Buffer
c.	**Probiotic**	d.	Oxidant

87. The colour of good silage should be:

a.	Green	b.	Red
c.	Brown	**d.**	**Light brown**

88. Green fodder is best source of:

a.	**Fat soluble vitamin**	b.	Protein
c.	Water soluble vitamin	d.	Lipid

89. Indicate laxative feed among the following:

a.	Crushed maize	b.	Crushed barley
c.	Crushed gram	**d.**	**Wheat bran**

90. Indicate which feed is highest in energy content among the following:

a.	**Maize**	b.	Ground nut meal
c.	Cotton seed meal	d.	Sal seed meal

91. Ground nut straw contains:

a. 4.5 % CP
b. 5.5 % CP
c. 3.0 % CP
d. 8.3 % CP

92. The ideal moisture percentage of hay making is:

a. 12-15 %
b. 15-18 %
c. 20-25 %
d. 25-30 %

93. The pH of good silage is:

a. 3.5 - 4.0
b. 4.2 – 4.5
c. 4.5 – 4.8
d. 4.8 – 6.8

94. Teosinte is a fodder crop of:

a. Rabi season
b. Kharif season
c. Zaid season
d. Both b & c

95. Cereal grains are rich in:

a. TDN and net energy
b. Calcium
c. Lysine
d. DCP

96. Number of essential amino acid in animal feeding:

a. 5
b. 10
c. 15
d. 20

97. Wheat straw contains:

a. 20 % TDN
b. 30 % TDN
c. 40 % TDN
d. 50 % TDN

98. Deficiency of iron in piglet causes:

a. Swine fever
b. Rickets
c. Polyneuritis
d. Anaemia

99. Another name of vitamin C is:

a. Thiamine
b. Ascorbic acid
c. Riboflavin
d. Cyanocobalamin

100. Which of the following should not be fed urea:

a. Bull b. Heifers

c. Calf d. Cow

101. Indicate which feed is highest in DCP:

a. Mustard cake **b. Ground nut cake**

c. Till cake d. Lin seed cake

102. Flowering stage of green fodder is having:

a. Low protein b. Medium protein

c. Rich protein d. No protein

103. The micro-organism used for the treatment of poor quality roughages:

a. Bacteria b. Virus

c. Protozoa **d. Fungus**

104. Yellow maize grain contains:

a. Vitamin A b. Vitamin B

c. Vitamin D_3 **d. Carotene**

105. Cotton seed contains toxic principle called:

a. Dicoumarol b. Hydrogen cyanide

c. Gossypol d. Lathyrus

106. Ammonia gas is used for the treatment of roughages to :

a. Improved digestibility

b. Increase nitrogen content

c. Improve nitrogen content and digestibility

d. Improve mineral content

107. The vitamins which contain sulphur are:

a. Thiamine and biotin b. Riboflavin and thiamine

c. Biotin and choline d. Choline and riboflavin

108. The proteolytic enzymes secreted from pancreas are:

a. Pepsin, trypsin and chymotrypsin

b. Trypsin, chymotrypsin and carboxypeptidase

c. Pepsin, chymotrypsin and carboxypeptidase

d. Pepsin, trypsin and carboxypeptidase

109. The net ATP production from one mole of acetic acid is:

a.	17 moles	b.	25 moles
c.	**10 moles**	d.	12 moles

110. The amino acids which do not participate in transmutation:

a.	Lysine and histidine	b.	Lysine and methionine
c.	Lysine and tryptophan	**d.**	**Lysine and threonine**

111. Which one of the following is a rumen protozoa:

a. ***Dasytricha ruminantium***

b. *Selenomonas ruminantium*

c. *Megasphaera elsdenii*

d. *Methanobacterium ruminantium*

112. The calcium content in the animal body is:

a.	**1.33 %**	b.	0.33 %
c.	3.33 %	d.	7.33 %

113. In all roughage diet the dominant volatile fatty acid in cattle is:

a.	Propionic acid	b.	Butyric acid
c.	**Acetic acid**	d.	Formic acid

114. Depigmentation of colour hair and black wool is a common finding in:

a.	Iron deficiency	**b.**	**Copper deficiency**
c.	Magnesium deficiency	d.	Calcium deficiency

115. Which of the following is protein supplement for livestock:

a.	Cereals	b.	Cereal byproduct
c.	Non leguminous roughage	**d.**	**Oilcake**

116. Instrument used for grinding of feed ingredients:

a.	Roller mill	b.	Attrition and burr mill
c.	Hammer mill	**d.**	**All of the above**

117. One calorie is equal to:

a. 0.293 joule
b. 0.239 joule
c. 4.184 joule
d. 3.601 joule

118. *Leucaena leucocephala* contains anti nutritional factor as:

a. Oxalate
b. Gossypol
c. Glucosinolates
d. Mimosine

119. When a substance is completely burned to its ultimate oxidation product i.e. carbon dioxide, water and other gases, the heat given off is considered as its:

a. Gross energy
b. Digestible energy
c. Metabolisable energy
d. Net energy

120. Practically any crop having sufficient soluble carbohydrates and moisture to produce desired quantities of acids may be made into:

a. Hay
b. Silage
c. Both of the above
d. None of the above

121. To arrive at the metabolisable energy of feed, the digestible energy is multipled by the factor:

a. 0.99
b. 0.96
c. 0.82
d. 0.76

122. To arrive the TDN value of feed the % DEE is multiplied by the:

a. 5.25
b. 1.25
c. 3.25
d. 2.25

123. Which is the main product(s) of protein digestion in animals:

a. Acetic acid
b. Amino acids
c. Alkali
d. Atomic energy

124. The main products of carbohydrate digestion in the rumen are:

a. Vermicides
b. Vinyl ether
c. Vitamins
d. Volatile fatty acids

125. A major portion of phosphorus in the animal body is found in:

a. Blood b. Brain

c. Bones d. Body fluids

126. Sodium chloride deficiency in poultry leads to the condition called:

a. Cannibalism b. Chlorination

c. Catabolism d. Chelating

127. Ground limestone is added in the rations of livestock & poultry to supply:

a. Iron b. Sodium

c. Magnesium **d. Calcium**

128. Glycogen synthesis from simple sugars in the body tissues is known as:

a. Gluconeogenesis b. Glycogenolysis

c. Glycogenesis d. Glycolysis

129. Crude protein in feedstuffs is estimated by multiplying nitrogen content with a factor:

a. 5.25 b. 6.00

c. 6.25 d. 6.50

130. The ether extract is that fraction of the feedstuffs which is obtained on continuous extraction of the material with:

a. Acids b. Alkali

c. Water **d. Petroleum ether**

131. Crude protein content in a good quality cottonseed meal is around:

a. 20 % b. 30 %

c. 40 % d. 50 %

132. Which of these is an incriminating factor found in cottonseed meal:

a. Saponin b. Sinapin

c. Gossypol d. Waxpol

133. Good quality rapeseed meal contains crude protein around:

a. 20% b. 30%

c. 40% d. 50%

134. One of the important antinutritional component found in rapeseed meal is:

a. Galactose
b. Glucose
c. Glycogen
d. Glucosinolate

135. Which one of the following is a feedstuff of choice as an energy source in pig feeding:

a. Masoor
b. Milo
c. Maize
d. Mustard cake

138. For estimation of crude protein in feedstuffs which of the following elements is determined:

a. Neptunium
b. Niobicom
c. Nitrogen
d. Nobelium

139. Which of the following elements is absent in lipids:

a. Carbon
b. Hydrogen
c. Nitrogen
d. Oxygen

140. The ingredient of choice as calcium supplement in poultry feeding is:

a. Calcium hydroxide
b. Calcium iodate
c. Calcium carbonate
d. Calcium sulphate

141. Physiological fuel value of fat (Kcal/gm) is:

a. 9.4
b. 9.2
c. 9.0
d. 9.15

142. The digestion mixture in crude protein estimation consists of:

a. Copper sulphate and potassium sulphate
b. Copper sulphate and sodium hydroxide
c. Potassium sulphate and sodium hydroxide
d. All of the above

143. The minerals that play most important role in osmotic regulation of body fluids are:

a. Na^+ K^+ and Cl^-
b. Na^+ K^+ and S^+
c. Na^+ Mg^+ and K^+
d. Na^+ Mg^+ and Mn^+

144. Perosis in chicken is caused by deficiency of:

a. Zinc
b. Iodine
c. Magnesium
d. Manganese

145. The vitamin which acts as a hormone is:

a. Vit. A
b. Vit. D
c. Vit. E
d. Vit. K

146. In ruminants, the end products of carbohydrate fermentation are:

a. Acetate, propionate and butyrate
b. Acetate, citrate and valerate
c. Acetate, succinate and oxaloacetate
d. Acetate, butyrate and oxalosuccinate

147. The ingredient that is rich in phosphorus is:

a. Shell grit
b. Dicalcium phosphate
c. Lime stone
d. Calcite

148. The commonly used antioxidant in compound feeds is:

a. Aureomycin
b. EDTA
c. BHT
d. Zinc sulphate

149. Oxalates found in some fodder crops from insoluble complexes with:

a. Zinc
b. Magnesium
c. Calcium
d. Phosphorous

150. Which one of the following is a leguminous fodder crop:

a. Sorghum
b. Cluster bean
c. Maize
d. Oat

151. The moisture content of a hay should not exceed:

a. 15 %
b. 20 %
c. 10 %
d. 25 %

152. IN NRC feeding standard, the energy requirements for swine are expressed as:

a. Digestible energy
b. Gross energy
c. Net energy
d. TDN

153. Zearalenone is a mycotoxin produced by:

a. *Aspergillus* spp. b. *Penicillium* spp.

c. *Fusarium* spp. d. *Eubacterium* spp.

154. Star gazing is a condition seen in chicks due to the deficiency of:

a. Riboflavin b. Pantothenic acid

c. Vit. A **d. Thiamine**

155. Falling disease is a condition seen in:

a. Cattle b. Calves and lambs

c. Camel d. Pigs

156. Which of the following combination is grouped under non nutrient feed additives:

a. Dried rumen culture, folic acid and zinc

b. Coccidiostats, dried rumen culture and hormones

c. Manganese, biotin and vitamin K

d. Methionine, sulfur and biotin

157. The ideal Ca:P ratio in the diet of the most of the livestock should be:

a. 1:1 b. 1:2

c. 2:1 d. 1:4

158. Mobilization of calcium from bone take place under the influence of:

a. Parathormone **b. Calcitonin**

c. STH d. ACTH

159. Consumption of raw egg may produce the deficiency of:

a. Choline **b. Biotin**

c. Niacin d. Thiamin

160. In poultry nutritional roup is caused by the deficiency of:

a. Vitamin K **b. Vitamin A**

c. Vitamin E d. Vitamin B

161. Enlargement of hock joint is seen due to the deficiency of:

a. Selenium b. Manganese

c. Zinc d. Potassium

162. The green forages which are cut and fed in fresh condition to the animals are termed as:

a. Green fodder b. Silage

c. Green grass d. Sialage

163. Feed stuffs which are very rich in NFE and TDN but low in CF (generally less than 18%) are referred to us:

a. Energy feeds **b. Concentrates**

c. Silages d. Feed additives

164. Cotton seed meal is usually not recommended in the chickens as it contains a glycoside:

a. linamarine b. Cynogenic glycoside

c. Gossypol d. Hipuric acid

165. One gram of fat produces how much gram of metabolic water on its complete oxidation:

a. 0.64 b. 0.42

c. 1.1 d. 0.84

166. One gram of TDN provides Kcal of ME:

a. 4.41 **b. 3.65**

c. 4.00 d. 3.85

169. In a normal feeding regimen cow produces methane which results in loss of energy to the tune of:

a. 15 % of GE b. 20 % of GE

c. 7 % of GE d. 13 % of GE

170. One hundred gram of carbohydrate metabolism produces how many grams of metabolic water:

a. 40 **b. 60**

c. 0.6 d. None of the above

171. Butyric acid metabolism produces moles of ATP:

a. 17 b. 27

c. 10 **d. None of the above**

172. Which one is sulphur containing amino acid:

a. Tyrosine b. Citrulline

c. Methionine d. Glycine

173. Which one is saturated fatty acid:

a. Oleic acid **b. Stearic acid**

c. Archidonic acid d. All of the above

174. Pica (deprived appetite) is specific deficiency of mineral:

a. Magnesium b. Potassium

c. Phosphorus d. All of the above

175. Wool is the deficiency symptoms of mineral:

a. Potassium b. Cobalt

c. Zinc **d. None of the above**

176. Which of the following feed ingredients is not a protein supplement:

a. Soybean meals b. Groundnut cake

c. **Maize grain** d. None of the above

177. The factor for calculating protein in milk from nitrogen is:

a. 6.25 **b. 6.38**

c. 5.75 d. 6.75

178. The respiratory quotient (R.Q.) of carbohydrates is:

a. 1.0 b. 0.90

c. 0.70 d. None of the above

179. Aflatoxin is a:

a. Fungal toxin b. Bacterial toxin

c. Viral toxin d. All of the above

180. Gross energy of one gram fat is:

a. 4.09 kcal
b. 4.90 kcal
c. 9.4 kcal
d. 9.04 kcal

181. Unripe potato contains an anti nutritional factor:

a. Quinine
b. Strychnine
c. Solanine
d. Nicotine

182. One kilogram of digestible starch produces fats is:

a. 248 g
b. 235 g
c. 268 g
d. 474 g

183. Which of the following is an essential fatty acid for poultry:

a. Arachidonic acid
b. Caproic acid
c. Butyric acid
d. Erucic acid

184. Which one of the following amino acids contain sulphur in its molecule:

a. Arginine
b. Cystine
c. Glutamic acid
d. Leucine

185. In poultry, black tongue disease is caused by the deficiency of:

a. Nitrogen
b. Nucleic acids
c. Niacin
d. Nitrates

186. Which one of the followings is used in diet of farm livestock to prevent phosphorus deficiency:

a. Phosphomin
b. Dicalcium phosphate
c. Phosphoric acid
d. Fluorine

187. Ruminants are able to utilize dietary cellulose with the help of:

a. Pectinase
b. Lipase
c. Microbial cellulase enzymes
d. Protease

188. Which of the following enzymes aids in protein digestion:

a. Lipase
b. Pepsin
c. Cellulase
d. Hemicellulase

189. Which of the following is the end product of amino acid deamination in poultry:

a.	**Uric acid**	b.	Uronic acid
c.	Uracil	d.	Urea

190. The physiological fuel value for one gram protein has been calculated at:

a.	**4.00**	b.	4.15
c.	5.65	d.	9.40

191. Calcium content in pure feed grade limestone should be around:

a.	30.0 %	b.	36.0 %
c.	**39.0 %**	d.	45.0 %

192. Mango seed kernel has poor nutritive value for the non-ruminants due to being fairly rich in:

a.	Silica	b.	Lignin
c.	**Tannins**	d.	Mowrine

193. Crude protein content in a good quality soybean meal is around:

a.	25 %	b.	30 %
c.	**45 %**	d.	65 %

194. One of the important deleterious substance in guar meal is:

a.	Glucosinolate	**b.**	**Guar Gum**
c.	Ricin	d.	Mowrin

195. Which of the followings is energy feed of choice for fattening pigs:

a.	Salseed meal	b.	Guar meal
c.	Linseed meal	**d.**	**Maize**

196. Green berseem is a good source of:

a.	Vitamin E	b.	Vitamin A
c.	Vitamin D	**d.**	**Carotene**

197. Subabul makes a good fodder for the ruminants but it should not be fed to pigs and horses due to the presence of a toxic amino acid:

a.	Lysine	**b.**	**Mimosine**
c.	Methionine	d.	Leuecine

198. The composition of rumen gases is:

a. CO_2 and H_2 b. CO_2 and CH_4

c. CO_2, H_2 and CH_4 d. H_2 and CH_4

199. Oxidation of one mole of glucose to CO_2 and water yields mole of ATP:

a. 8 b. 28

c. 38 d. 28

200. More commonly used factor for converting nitrogen to crude protein:

a. 5.25 b. 4.25

c. 6.75 **d. 6.25**

201. Ruminants meet their major energy requirement from:

a. Glucose b. Pyruvate

c. Volatile fatty acids d. Microbial protein

202. A shift from high concentrate diet to high roughage diet increases the production of:

a. Acetic acid b. Butyric acid

c. Propionate d. None of the above

203. The simplest sugars are the:

a. Disaccharides **b. Monosaccharide**

c. Trisaccharides d. None of the above

204. A fat soluble vitamin is:

a. Choline b. Biotin

c. Phylloquinone **d. Folacin**

205. Urea may be added in the diet of:

a. Pets b. Poultry

c. Sheep d. Pig

206. Plants cell wall is mainly composed of:

a. Cellulose and hemicellulose

b. Cellulose and lignin

c. **Cellulose, hemicellulose and lignin**

d. Hemicellulose and lignin

207. Fats provide how many times higher energy than carbohydrates:

a. 1.25 b. 2.50

c. 2.25 d. 2.55

208. Which of the following is included in the ration as protein supplement:

a. Rice polish b. Wheat bran

c. Sorghum **d. Soybean meal**

209. Rice straw contain (%TDN and DCP) respectively:

a. 0.00 & 40 **b. 40 & 0.00**

c. 4.00 & 60 d. 60 & 4.00

210. Which of the following is used as roughage source in ruminant's diet:

a. Wheat straw b. Wheat bran

c. Corn gluten meal d. Linseed meal

211. Which of the following fatty acid is responsible for milk fat synthesis in cow?

a. Acetic acid b. Butyric acid

c. Propionate d. Pentothenic acid

212. A polysaccharide in animal body is:

a. Starch b. Cellulose

c. Glycogen d. Dextrin

213. Biological value of protein is primarily dependent upon:

a. NPN content **b. Indispensable amino acid**

c. Glycogen level d. Uric acid content

214. Urea treatment of roughages improves their:

a. Intake b. Utilization

c. Intake and utilization d. None of the above

Q.3. Fill in the Blanks :

1. Animal body contains ***40 to 65 %*** water.
2. "Egg white injury" is caused by ***avidine*** which prevents absorption of ***biotin.***

3. Swayback is due to deficiency of ***copper*** in ***lambs***.
4. Polyneuritis is due to deficiency of ***thiamine*** in ***chicks.***
5. Black tongue is due to deficiency of ***niacin*** in ***dog.***
6. Metabolism of protein yields ***40%*** of its weight as metabolic water.
7. Vitamin dietary essential for ruminants is ***vitamin A.***
8. Naturally occurring free form of vitamin B_6 are ***pyridoxine and pyridoxal***
9. Spontaneous combustion is occasionally seen in ***hay*** making.
10. Concentrates contain less than ***18%*** crude fibre and more than ***60%*** TDN.
11. Natural toxicant present in cotton seed cake is known as ***gossypol***.
12. Heat increment includes ***HF*** and ***HNM.***
13. Good quality hay should contain <***15%*** moisture.
14. Predominant acid in good quality silage is ***lactic acid.***
15. Optimum level of formaldehyde for protection of concentrate protein is ***3 percent.***
16. Conversion of carotene to vitamin A occurs mainly in ***intestine wall***.
17. Rickets is caused due to the deficiency of ***calcium enzyme***.
18. Cellulose is most impervious to ***enzyme*** digestion.
19. Cynogenetic glycosides liberate ***HCN*** on hydrolysis.
20. Goiter is caused due to the deficiency of ***iodine***
21. Curled toe paralysis takes place in poultry due to the deficiency of ***riboflavin.***
22. Digestibility of protozoal protein is ***91*** percent.
23. Pantothenic acid deficiencies have been reported in ***landrace*** pig herds.
24. Fat content of rice polish is about ***12 percent.***
25. The water content of concentrates should be about ***10percent.***
26. The losses of dry matter by white rot fungal treatment for straw goes upto ***25 percent.***
27. Poor quality roughages generally contain ***48 %*** TDN.
28. The crude protein content of ground nut cake is about ***45 percent.***
29. Fish meal contains ***9.3%*** nitrogen.

30. Most indigestible cementing material present alongwith cellulose and hemicellulose in plants is ***lignin.***

31. Cellulose is a polymer of ***beta glucose.***

32. Lignin is most impervious to ***enzyme*** digestion.

33. Oxidative phosphorylation takes place within ***mitochondria.***

34. Conversion of carotene to vitamin A takes place mainly in ***intestinal wall.***

35. Pantothenic acid can be produced by the bacteria ***E.coli.***

36. Grass tetany is caused due to manifestation of ***magnesium*** deficiency.

37. Oilseeds are generally rich sources of ***essential fatty*** acid.

38. Ash is the inorganic residue estimated after burning the feed sample at ***600ºC***

39. The losses of silages in kachcha pit may go upto ***20*** percent.

40. Metabolizable energy represents about ***41%*** of the gross energy in hay feeding.

41. Methane contains ***13.34*** Kcal per gm.

42. The BV of microbial proteins is ***80*** percent.

43. The excretion of nitrogen in the faeces is known as ***MFN.***

44. Two German scientists associated with Weende method of analysis of feed are ***Henneberg and Stohmann.***

45. Starch consists of a mixture of two types of polymers ***amylase*** and ***amylopectins.***

46. The end products of cellulose digestion in ruminants are not sugars but ***VFA.***

47. Lipoproteins are common constituent of ***cell membrane*** in animals.

48. Molybdenum is an active mineral of the enzyme ***xanthine oxidase.***

49. Exudative diathesis in chicks is due to deficiency of mineral ***selenium.***

50. Propionate is converted to glucose by first entering the TCA cycle as ***succinyl co-A.***

51. All forms of energy can be quantitatively converted to ***heat energy.***

52. Cereal grains are generally deficient in essential amino acid ***lysine.***

53. Dominant acid in wall preserved silage is ***lactic acid.***

54. G.E.value of feeds can be determined in an instrument known as ***bomb calorimeter.***

55. Both chemical score and EAAT are based upon gross ***amino acid*** composition.

56. NE is the difference between ME and ***heat increment*** in ruminants.

57. A cereal grain contains very high NFE and CF content is low in ***maize.***

58. Iodine is a constituent of hormone ***thyroxine.***

59. Biological amines are formed by ***decarboxylation*** of amino acids.

60. Melting point of fatty acid ***increase*** as the chain length increases.

61. A French chemist ***Antoine Lavoisier*** referred to as the founder of science of nutrition.

62. In birds ***uric acid*** is the principle end product of nitrogen metabolism.

63. ***Glycine*** is the essential amino acid only for chicks.

64. B-carotene is a precursor of ***vit. A***.

65. One gram nitrogen is equivalent to ***6.5g*** CP.

66. A toxic substancc prcscnt in *Leucaena leucocephala* is ***mimosine.***

67. The form of energy that is stored in the plant is ***chemical energy.***

68. Heat increment is determined by the instrument known as ***respiration calorimeter.***

69. Starch equivalent (SE) system was developed by ***Oskar Kellner.***

70. Two mineral acids used in AIV silage are ***HCl and*** H_2So_4.

71. The apparent DE of a feed is the GE minus the energy contained in ***faeces.***

72. Alpha–amino Beta-imidazole propionic acid is ***histidine.***

73. Polymerized structure of polypeptide is referred as ***quarternary structure.***

74. Glycolipids are compounds occurring most commonly in ***nerve tissue.***

75. Fats are hydrolysed to ***glycerol*** and fatty acid by the action of enzyme ***lipase.***

76. Rumen content pH varies between ***5.5 to 6.5.***

77. The omasum is a spherical organ filled with muscular ***laminae.***
78. Glycerol's are fermented in the rumen and formed ***propionic acid.***
79. The sugar fermenting bacteria in the rumen is ***lacto bacilli***.
80. The cultivated forage and grasses when ensiled at higher dry matter content, the ensiled matter is termed as ***haylage.***
81. Hay should possess reasonably green colour which give a rough idea of ***chlorophyll*** the carotene.
82. Vitamin K activity is inhibited by ***dicoumarol compound.***
83. Alakali used for the treatment of poor quality roughages is ***sodium hydroxide.***
84. Molasses used as a cattle feed as a source of ***energy.***
85. Rice polish contains ***15-17 percent*** crude fat.
86. Increase quantities of sugar and starches in the diet decreases the concentration ***ammonia*** in the rumen.
87. The absorption of leucine and phenyl alanine is inhibited by ***methionine.***
88. Dietary protein is degraded at different rates but often rapidly by ***microbial*** action in the rumen.
89. The polysaccharide stored in the animal body is ***glycogen.***
90. ***Pinocytosis*** is a passive transport system of nutrient in gastro-intestinal tract.
91. Fats are digested in gastro-intestinal tract in ***alkaline*** medium.
92. Biotin is a part of acyl coenzyme-A ***carboxylase.***
93. Tree leaves are rich in calcium content but poor in ***phosphorus*** content.
94. Ground nut cake used as a supplement of ***protein*** in the diet.
95. Urea is hydrolysed in the rumen to ***ammonia*** and carbon dioxide.
96. Nutriture refers to the ***nutritional status*** of the animal.
97. A metal required for the synthesis of vitamin B_{12} in ruminants is ***cobalt.***
98. ***Antoine Lavoisier*** is a French chemist who is commonly referred to as the father of nutrition.
99. In young calvcs thc coagulation of milk proteins takes place due to the action of enzyme ***rennin.***

100. For horses the principal organs of prehension are ***lips.***

101. Perosis or slipped tendon in birds is caused due to deficiency of ***manganese*** mineral.

102. Roughages generally contain more than ***18%*** crude fibre and less than ***60%*** TDN.

103. Losses of soluble nutrients in hay due to rainwater are known as ***leaching.***

104. The formula for calculating TDN is TDN %=***DCP%+DCF%+DNFE%+ 2.25 DEE%.***

105. In proximate analysis of feed, the fraction of feed that is not chemically estimated, but arrived at by difference is known as ***nitrogenous free extract*** (NFE).

106. Tree leaves in general are rich in anti nutritional factor known as ***tannins.***

107. Net energy is the difference between metabolisable energy and ***heat*** increment in ruminants.

108. Animal proteins have ***higher/more*** biological values than plant proteins.

109. In Scandinavian feed unit system ***barley*** (cereal) have been taken as standard unit.

110. Chemical compounds which may be converted into vitamins in the body are known as ***provitamins and vitamin precursors.***

111. Choline deficiency in poultry is generally associated withy a condition called ***perosis or slipped tendon.***

112. Phosphorus deficiency in diet of adult animals leads to a condition called ***osteomalacia.***

113. In dairy herds, deficiency of magnesium has been characterized by the names like ***grass tetany / magnesium tetany.***

114. Abnormal wool growth in sheep is observed due to the deficiency of ***copper.***

115. Cobalt is needed by the rumen micro-organisms for synthesis of ***vitamin*** B_{12}***/cyanocobalamine.***

116. Zinc deficiency in pigs leads to a condition referred to as ***parakeratosis.***

117. Sweet clover disease in cattle is caused due to presence of a compound ***dicoumarol*** which lowers the prothrombin level in blood.

118. In a feedstuff, the crude protein is estimated by determining the ***nitrogen*** content.

119. The nitrogen excreted through the faecal material is from both the undigested feed and also of ***metabolic*** origin.

120. The respiratory quotient is the ratio between the volume of carbon dioxide produced by the animal and the volume of the ***oxygen*** used.

121. Digestibility of low grade roughages can be improved through treatment with ***alkali.***

122. Protein efficiency ratio is defined as body weight gain per unit of ***protein*** intake.

123. Concentrate feeds are less bulky and contain less than ***18%*** crude fiber.

124. For efficient production of good quality hay, moisture content in the green crop is reduced to ***20%*** or even lesser.

125. Carrot is a rich source of ***carotene.***

126. Maltose on hydrolysis yields two molecules of ***glucose.***

127. ***Pantothenic acid*** is called as vitamin B_5.

128. ***Casimir Funk*** coined the term vitamin.

129. ***Oleic acid*** is a monounsaturated fatty acid, while ***linoleic acid*** is an unsaturated fatty acid.

130. The net gain of ATP from one mole or glucose in aerobic glycolysis is ***8.***

131. ***Diethylstilbestrol*** is a hormone commonly used as implants in beef cattle to enhance body weight gain.

132. Protein equivalent of urea is ***260-280* percent.**

133. Fibre fractionation was developed by ***Van Soest.***

134. ***Bomb calorimeter*** is the instrument used to estimate gross energy of a feedstuff.

135. Indian feeding standards are based on ***Morrison*** feeding standards.

136. ***DCP/bone meal/fish meal*** is a phosphorus rich feed ingredient.

137. One kg TDN is equivalent to ***4.4 mcal*** of digestible energy.

138. ***Fish meal and meat meal*** are examples of animal protein feed ingredients.

139. ***Dicoumarol*** is responsible for sweet clover disease.

140. Soybean is a rich source of ***metheonine*** amino acid.

141. Selenium is the component of ***glutathione oxidase*** enzyme system.

142. A newly recognized essential trace element required for the synthesis of mucopolysaccharide is ***silicon.***

143. Pica is caused due to dietary deficiency of ***phosphorus*** in dairy animals.

144. The energy equivalent of EE is about ***2.25 times of carbohydrate***.

145. A feed rich in digestible protein in proportion to non nitrogenous nutrients have ***narrow*** nutritive ratio.

146. The determination of proximate principles of feed was first proposed by the scientist ***Henneberg.***

147. On a fat and moisture free basis animal body contain ***80*** percent protein.

148. Young animals have ***higher*** water needs per unit of body size than mature animals.

149. The simplest sugar is ***monosaccharides*** which cannot be hydrolyzed into smaller units under mild conditions.

150. All proteins contain on an average about ***16*** percent of nitrogen.

151. Fatty acid containing more than one double bond is called ***polyunsaturated fatty acid.***

152. The active forms of vitamin D are ***ergocalciferol and cholecalciferol***.

153. After removal of starch and germ from maize, the product obtained is called ***maize glutein.***

154. ***Leguminous*** type of fodder is best for hay making.

155. The container used for silage making is called ***silo.***

156. The term starch equivalent is given by ***Kellner.***

157. Protein efficiency ratio is the weight gain per unit of ***protein intake.***

158. The treatment of grains with direct flame is called ***roasting.***

159. Molasses is used in commercial pelleted feed as ***binder.***

160. Chemically speaking, fats are esters of fatty acids and ***glycerol.***

161. Amino acids contain both an amino group and a ***carboxyl*** group.

162. In young animals vit. D deficiency leads to the development of bone abnormality called ***rickets.***

163. In retina of eye, vitamin A combines with a protein to form visual purple called ***rhodopsin.***

164. Certain closely related chemical compounds possessing vitamin E activity are known by ***tocopherols.***

165. Iodine deficiency in farm livestock can be prevented through the feeding of ***iodised*** salts.

166. The deficiency of ***cobalt*** element is responsible for insufficient synthesis of vitamin B_{12} by the rumen microorganisms.

167. Indirect calorimetric studies for energy metabolism on farm animals an apparatus called ***respiration chamber*** is used for this purpose.

168. Sorghum grains are less palatable than maize due to the presence of chemical compounds called ***tannins*** in them.

169. Full fat rice polish is rich in energy and also a good source of many of the ***B complex*** vitamins.

170. For non ruminants, soybean meal is fairly deficient in one of the essential amino acids named ***methionine.***

171. Guar seed is unique in that it is completely devoid of a polysaccharide ***starch*** usually found in seeds.

172. Improperly processed soybean meal shows high activity of the enzyme ***urease.***

173. Calcium is the most abundant mineral in the ***animal*** body.

174. Black tongue disease occurs due to the efficiency of ***nicotinic acid.***

175. Rickets is a condition which occurs due to dietary deficiency of ***vitamin D.***

176. Chicks reared on a ***riboflavin*** deficient diet grow slowly and develop curled toe paralysis.

177. Vitamin A is chemically known as ***retinol.***

178. 1, 25-dihydroxycholecalciferol is the most biological active form of ***vitamin D.***

179. ***Alkali/Degnala*** disease occurs due to the toxicity of selenium.

180. Biological value is the proportion of the N absorbed and ***retained*** in the animal.

181. Silage is good substitute for ***green forage.***

182. Mimosine is an ***antinutritional*** factor present in subabul (*Lucaenea leucocephala*).

183. Cotton seed cake is a good source of ***protein.***

184. Hay making is done to reduce the ***moisture*** content of green crops.

7

Animal Nutrition (Part-II) Applied Nutrition of Livestock, Human Pets & other Animals

Q.1. Write "True" or "False" Against Each Statement

1. True — Feeding of large quantities of legumes may lead to phosphorous deficiency.
2. True — Daily water requirement of hen is approximately double the quantity of dry matter intake.
3. True — Feeding of too much hay or greens reduces the breeding ability of bulls.
4. False — Generally urea is not fed more than 1.0% of the total dry matter intake.
5. True — A cow needs about 3.5 kg water for every kg of milk produced.
6. False — The maintenance requirement of a cow varies with her metabolic body size.
7. False — About 15 g of protein is required daily by a laying hen for egg production and maintenance.
8. True — Supplementary feeding of infants should be started from 4 months.
9. True — Carbohydrates yield metabolic water to the tune of 60 percent.
10. True — An adolescent girl requires minimum quantity of iron.
11. True — Vitamin A helps in the absorption of calcium and phosphorus.

12. True — Dry method of cooking results in greater loss of nutrients than wet method.

13. True — The first limiting amino acid in cereal grains is lysine.

14. True — Lactose and sucrose are poorly digested in dog.

15. True — The deficiency of iodine in human beings may lead to cretinism.

16. True — The chemical analysis of feeds does not give the information about availability of nutrients present in the feeding stuffs to the animals.

17. True — The basic principle involved in digestion trial is measuring the quantities of nutrients consumed and the quantities of nutrients excreted in faeces during an experimental period.

18. False — In indirect system of digestibility determination only one digestibility trial is conducted.

19. True — In indicator method of digestibility determination the index or indicator substances are either consumed by the animals in the feed or are administered to the animals.

20. False — Total digestible nutrients (TDN)=% digestible crude protein+%digestible crude fiber+% digestible NFE+% digestible ether extract.

21. True — The biological value of protein is defined as the percentage of absorbed protein which is utilized by the body.

22. False — The maintenance requirements of non-producing animals are stated as the amount of nutrients sufficient to maintain the body weight besides maintaining normal physiological functions under working conditions.

23. False — The birds are able to adjust the energy requirement by voluntary intake of feed. The feed intake of the growing chicken will in general increase as the energy content of the ration is increased.

24. False — The dietary habits of human in different region of world have been determined by the local availability of foods and well taken care of all nutrients requirement of the persons living in that region.

25. False — There are about twenty amino acids commonly found in dietary proteins and required by the body. Out of them twelve amino acids cannot be synthesized by the body and hence have to be supplied through the diet. These amino acids are called 'essential amino acids'.

26. True — The gain in weight of young animals per unit of protein consumed is measured and the value thus obtained is known as the 'protein efficiency ratio'.

27. False — Vitamin B_6 is also called cyanocobalamin.

28. False — Vitamin C is the vitamin that prevents a condition called 'beri-beri'.

29. False — A very cheap and common fruit, namely 'Amla' (*Phyllanthus emblica*) is very rich in vitamin D.

30. True — The DCP requirement for maintenance of a 400 kg cow is 254 gm.

31. False — The poultry starts laying at 12 weeks of age.

32. True — Example of natural marker is lignin.

33. False — Digestibility of concentrates is estimated by indicator method.

34. False — In poultry ration generally fish meal is added at 20% level.

35. True — Urea can be included in cows ration at the rate of 1% of DM.

36. False — Collection period in conventional digestion trial is of 15 days.

37. False — Wheat is a pellagrogenic food.

38. False — Milk is a stable food.

39. False — Red fiery tongue indicates deficiency of thiamine.

40. False — Riboflavin plays its role in the metabolism through TPP.

41. False — Cats do not require taurine in their diet.

42. False — Dogs have higher requirement of animal protein than cats.

43. True — Coprophagy is normal habit in rabbits.

44. False — Group feeding data are much more used from the stand point of statistical treatments as compared to individual feeding.

45. False "Associative effect" of feed as observed in digestibility determination is more pronounced in non-ruminants than the ruminant animals.

46. False Voluntary feed intake in healthy adult cattle fed wheat straw a sole feed is about 3% of its body weight.

47. False Rice husk is quite palatable to ruminants.

48. True Botanical name of siris is *Albezia lebbeck.*

49. False Cattle manure generally contains more nitrogen per unit weight basis as compared to poultry.

50. True Maize gluten meal is fed to animals as a protein supplement.

51. True As per NRC (1998), the crude protein requirement in the diet for 3-5 kg body weight piglet is 26 percent.

52. False Taurine is not an end product of sulphur containing amino acid metabolism.

53. True Guinea pig requires vitamin C as dietary requirement.

54. True Feeding of mouldy hay to horse may cause respiratory problem.

55. False Diet containing more amounts of unsaturated fatty acids is less susceptible to rancidity.

56. True Cereal by-product is generally rich in phosphorus.

57. True Feeding of excess cereal reduces the bioavailability of phosphorus.

58. False Colostrum is the poor source of antibody and vitamin A.

59. True Faeces and urine samples are collected in a metabolic trial.

60. True Indicator method of determining digestibility can be used to determine the pasture consumption.

61. True For 1kg milk production of (4% fat) the cows require 46 gm of DCP.

62. True Methionine is the first limiting amino acid in soybean protein.

63. False Soybean contains a toxic substance known as linamarine.

64. True Sulphur containing amino acids are very important for wool production.

65. False — Cereals are deficient in methionine.

66. False — Cats require a dietary source of carotene.

67. True — Blood glucose level of human being is 80-100 mg/dl.

68. False — Vitamin C is dietary essential for dogs.

69. False — The CP content of rabbit ration should be 10 percent.

70. True — Vitamin A is stable during wet cooking.

71. True — Oedema is a characteristic symptom of kwashiorkor.

72. True — In infant diet 30% of total calories must be supplied through fats.

73. True — Colostrum is a rich source of globulins.

74. False — Roughage contains less fibre than concentrate.

75. False — Shell grits are used as a source of phosphorus for poultry.

76. True — Digestibility of feed is influenced by the species and age of the animals.

77. False — B-complex vitamins are dietary essential for adult ruminants.

78. True — Urea contains 46.6% nitrogen.

79. True — Cotton seed cake feeding results in hard butter fat production in dairy cattle.

80. False — As feed additives, antibiotics are more effective under clean managemental conditions.

81. True — Feed intake is released to the energy density of the diet.

82. False — Human milk is a good source of iron and vitamin D.

83. True — *Clostridium botulinum* is responsible for spoilage of canned foods and is highly toxic.

84. True — Most of the vitamin B-complex requirements in rabbits are met through coprophagy.

85. False — Guinea pig is a monogastric carnivore.

86. True — At 8 weeks of age, pups can be fed the same feed as that of mature dogs.

87. True — A source of vitamin D is essential for infants receiving unfortified milk and milk products.

88.	True	In chronic liver diseases and ascitis, feeding of high sodium feeds and common salt should be reduced drastically.
89.	True	The process of purification normally alters protein nature.
90.	False	The apparent and true digestibility will be same for a given diet.
91.	True	Energy density influences voluntary feed intake in monogastrics.
92.	True	TDN over estimates energy value of poor quality roughage.
93.	False	As per BIS, layer mash should contain 23% crude protein.
94.	True	Goats are lesser dependant on free water sources than other domestic livestock.
95.	True	Protein of cereals and pulses has a supplementary effect in human nutrition.
96.	False	Cholesterol is exclusively found in vegetable oils.
97.	True	Cat has higher protein requirement than dog.
98.	True	All the forage eaters (such as guinea pigs, horses, sheep, goat and cattle, rabbit) have the poorest ability to digest the fibre.
99.	False	LDL is less atherogenic than HDL.
100.	True	In contrast to rat, mouse and rabbit, the entire stomach of guinea pig is lined with glandular epithelium.
101.	True	Groundnut cake is poor in lysine.
102.	False	Lignin is an external indicator.
103.	False	The crude protein content of straw is more than that of hay.
104.	False	Lime stone is a good source of calcium and phosphorus.
105.	True	Urea enrichment of straw improves its protein content.
106.	False	Undecorticated oil cakes contain low crude fibre when compared to decorticated cakes.
107.	False	Legume hay is a poor source of calcium.
108.	True	There will be no added advantage of feeding antibiotic feed additives to adult cattle.

109. False The lactose content of human milk is less than that of cow's milk.

110. True Feeding of animal protein should be restricted during liver disorders in pet animals.

111. True Taurine is an essential amino acid for cat.

112. False Egg yolk is a poor source of iron.

113. False Guinea pigs do not require a dietary supply of vitamin C.

114. True Yeast is a good source of B-complex vitamins.

115. True The diet of obese dogs should be prepared from high fibre and low energy feeds.

116. False Energy requirements of pets decrease during fever.

117. True In paired feeding trial, the faster growing animals is penalized.

118. True Acetic acid can be used as antidote for urea poisoning.

119. False The efficiency of meat production is always higher than milk production in ruminants.

120. False The recommended calorie-protein ratio for layer is 155:1.

121. False True digestibility is always lower than apparent digestibility as it includes MFN losses.

122. True Methionine is the most limiting amino acid for wool growth.

123. True Casein is a purified source of protein.

124. False Calf starter and milk replacer are the same.

125. True Carbohydrate content of animal body is less than 1percent.

126. False Vitamin A is present as such in plants.

127. True The largest part of the protein in Indian human diet comes from cereals and pulses.

128. True Canned food for dogs is usually complete and balanced.

129. False Boiling increases curd tension of milk.

130. True Rabbits are basically herbivorous.

131. False Birth weight of buffalo calves in general is 15-20 kg.

132. False Calf starts nibbing usually from 6th week of age.

133. True — Steaming up process leads to production of stronger and heavier calves.

134. True — Daily maintenance requirement of DCP and TDN of buffalo heifer growing at the rate of 500 g/daily is 0.296 kg DCP and 3.64 kg TDN.

135. True — TDN content in green berseem is 12 percent.

136. True — In non-ruminants amino-acid requirements have been estimated from dose response relationship obtained by verifying the dietary supply of an individual amino acid and monitoring a production response.

137. True — Digestible crude protein requirement for milk production with 5% milk fat is 0.05 kg/kg milk yield.

138. True — A young rabbit below 20 weeks of age is called bunny.

139. True — The ME requirements of adult rabbit for maintenance is 125-130 Kcal/kg.

140. False — Growing rabbits require 300-500 ml of drinking water per kg metabolic body weight.

141. True — Lactating rabbit require 20-25% crude protein in the diet.

142. True — The length of caecum in rabbit is about 0.6 meter.

143. False — Pure beta-carotene is red in colour.

144. False — Alopecia and scaly skin around the eye are seen in the deficiency of riboflavin.

145. False — Carbonaceous feed are rich in DTP.

146. False — Energy requirement for maintenance can not be determined by C-N balance studies.

147. False — Animals grow at different rate but energy requirement is the same.

148. True — Wheat bran is a rich source of phosphorus.

149. False — Apparent digestibility of CP is less than true digestibility.

150. True — In general concentrates are feeds that are high in NFE and TDN but low in CF.

151. True — Diethylstilbestrol may improve NPN utilization in ruminants.

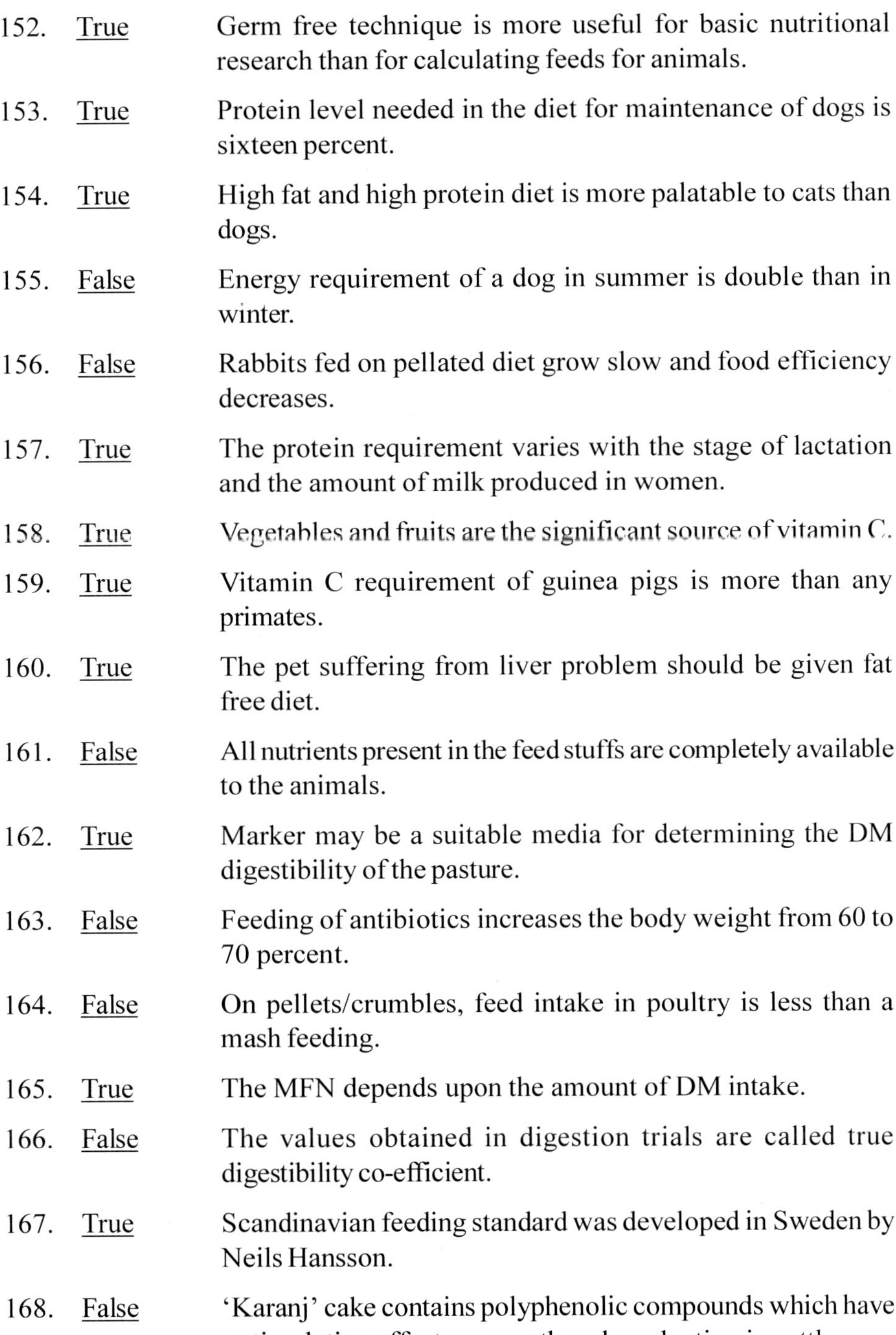

152. True — Germ free technique is more useful for basic nutritional research than for calculating feeds for animals.

153. True — Protein level needed in the diet for maintenance of dogs is sixteen percent.

154. True — High fat and high protein diet is more palatable to cats than dogs.

155. False — Energy requirement of a dog in summer is double than in winter.

156. False — Rabbits fed on pellated diet grow slow and food efficiency decreases.

157. True — The protein requirement varies with the stage of lactation and the amount of milk produced in women.

158. True — Vegetables and fruits are the significant source of vitamin C.

159. True — Vitamin C requirement of guinea pigs is more than any primates.

160. True — The pet suffering from liver problem should be given fat free diet.

161. False — All nutrients present in the feed stuffs are completely available to the animals.

162. True — Marker may be a suitable media for determining the DM digestibility of the pasture.

163. False — Feeding of antibiotics increases the body weight from 60 to 70 percent.

164. False — On pellets/crumbles, feed intake in poultry is less than a mash feeding.

165. True — The MFN depends upon the amount of DM intake.

166. False — The values obtained in digestion trials are called true digestibility co-efficient.

167. True — Scandinavian feeding standard was developed in Sweden by Neils Hansson.

168. False — ‘Karanj’ cake contains polyphenolic compounds which have a stimulating effect on growth and production in cattle.

169. False Digestibility of raw starch is high in dogs.

170. True Adult cats need 2g protein of biological value of 100% per kg body weight.

171. False Dogs confined to small pens generally require more energy than dogs permitted to exercise in large pens.

172. True Guinea pigs require high amount of ascorbic acid in the diet.

173. True Rats require all the 10 essential amino acids in the diet.

174. True The deficiency of iron occurs more in women than man.

175. True Vitamin E deficiency causes reproductive failure in cow.

176. True For the production of fatty carcass, cereal based energy rich feed is required.

177. False Lower lips of sheep split into two parts which help in grazing of grasses.

178. False Over feeding of milk should be avoided in calves otherwise it may cause tympanitis.

179. False The capacity of omasum in goat is about 3.0 liters.

180. Truc Mustard cake is not used in the diet of laboratory animals because of toxic compound present in it.

181. False Ground nut cake is used as energy source in the diet of guinea pigs.

182. False Bile is synthesized in the gall bladder and functions in the fat catabolism.

183. False Glycogen is a common ingredient of concentrate mixture of laboratory animals.

184. True About 10% of total phytate present in the diet are utilized by rat.

185. True Bran and oil cakes are rich source of magnesium.

186. True Vitamin A requirement of breeding rabbit is 8000 IU.

187. False Under stress condition feed conversion efficiency is always higher.

Q.2. Multiple Choices Questions :

1. Which one of the following is not suitable for poultry feeding:

   a. Mahua seed cake b. Soybean meal

   c. Peanut meal d. None of the above

2. An ideal calf starter should contain:

   A.18-20 % DCP and 75 % TDN

   b. 20-23 % DCP and 70 % TDN

   c. 24-25 % DCP and 75 % TDN

   d. 16-18 % DCP and 75 % TDN

3. For finishing goats complete ration should contain:

   a. 5-6 % DCP and 60-65 % TDN

   b. 8-10 % DCP and 60-65 % TDN

   c. 12-14 % DCP and 60-65 % TDN

   d. 16-18 % DCP and 60-65 % TDN

4. Complete development of rumen occurs at age of:

   a. 3 month b. 4 month

   c. 5 month **d. 6 month**

5. Creep ration is usually given to piglets when they attain the body weight of:

   a. 2 kg b. 4 kg

   c. 6 kg d. 8 kg

6. The calcium content of layer mash should be:

   a. 3% b. 4%

   c. 5% d. 6%

7. The most economical slaughter weight of pigs in Indian condition is:

   a. 60 kg b. 70 kg

   c. 80 kg d. 90 kg

8. Restricted feeding is practiced in birds in:

   a. Starters **b. Growers**

   c. Layers d. Breeders

9. The most potent carotenoid is:
   a. Beta carotene
   b. Alfa carotene
   c. Gamma carotene
   d. Cryptoxanthin

10. Fruits are very good source of:
   a. Potassium
   b. Calcium
   c. Magnesium
   d. Sodium

11. Which of the following is "Animal protein factor":
   a. Thiamine
   b. Riboflavin
   c. Pyridoxine
   d. Cyanocobalamine

12. Minimum nutrient loss during heat processing occurs in:
   a. Microwaving
   b. Freezing
   c. Drying
   d. Cooking

13. The casein: albumin ratio in human milk is:
   a. 1:1
   b. 3:1
   c. 5:1
   d. 7:1

14. The anti-sterility factor is:
   a. Vitamin A
   b. Vitamin E
   c. Selenium
   d. Glutathione peroxidase

15. Excess consumption of tea and coffee leads to:
   a. Indigestion
   b. Insomnia
   c. Constipation
   d. Bradycardia

16. Sweetest sugar is:
   a. Sucrose
   b. Fructose
   c. Glucose
   d. Lactose

17. The nitrogen which is excreted in the faeces even on a nitrogen free adequate diet is called :
   a. Endogerious unrinary nitrogen (EUN)
   b. Metabolic faecal nitrogen (MFN)
   c. Urinary nitrogen
   d. Total faecal nitrogen

18. The net yield of ATP obtained by the oxidation of per mole of propionic acid is:

a. 20 b. 19

c. 15 d. 18

19. There are certain compounds which are not themselve vitamins but function as vitamins only after undergoing a chemical change are called:

a. Antivitamins **b. Provitamins**

c. Prosthetic grounds d. Apoenzyme

20. In osteoporosis the mineral content of bone is normal but the absolute mass of bone is:

a. Increased b. Remain same

c. Reduced d. None of the above

21. Manganese deficiency in the diet of growing chicks is manifested as the disease:

a. Pica **b. Perosis**

c. Pigmentation failure d. Osteomalacia

22. Beri (*Zyziphus nummularia*) leaves are good source of protein (18.0%) but the digestibility is poor because of the presence of:

a. Saponins b. Gossypol

c. Tannins d. Lignin

23. Biological treatment of poor quality roughage is primarily done with the help of:

a. Bacteria b. Viruses

c. Fungi d. All of the above

24. Butylated hydroxytoluene (BHT) used as a feed additive in the diet of poultry comes under the category of:

a. Antibiotics b. Antifungals

c. Antioxidants d. Coccidiostate

25. Biot's spots or a white foamy patch which occur on the white portion of eyes is caused when diet does not contain adequate amount of:

a. Vitamin D b. Thiamine

c. Vitamin A d. Vitamin E

26. A protein-energy malnutrition marked by edema, peeling of skin into flakes, discoloration of hairs and irritability in children's is called:

    a. Scurvy **b. Kwashiorkor**
    c. Rickets d. Under-nutrition

27. Soreness and ulceration on lips and at the corners of mouth occuring due to deficiency of vitamin B-complex is termed as:

    a. Night blindness b. Rickets
    c. Chelosis d. Scurvery

28. The site of crude fiber digestion in rabbit is:

    a. Colon **b. Caecum**
    c. Small intestine d. Stomach

29. To maintain intestinal motility and avoid muco-entertis in rabbits, the requirement of crude fiber in the diet is:

    a. 5-8% b. 8-10%
    c. 10-15% d. 15-20%

30. To obtain best performance and production from rabbits one should feed rabbits with:

    a. Concentrate pellets and green fodder
    b. Complete pellets
    c. Concentrate mash and green fodder
    d. Kitchen wastes and green fodder

31. The requirement of crude protein in compound feed for guinea pig as per ISI recommended:

    a. 5% **b. 20-22%**
    c. 25% d. None of the above

32. The energy requirement of rats in their diet is:

    a. 3200 kcal ME/kg **b. 4000 kcal ME/kg**
    c. 2800 kcal ME/kg d. 2500 kcal ME/kg

33. Limiting amino acid in maize is:

    a. Tryptophan b. Methionine
    c. Lysine d. Arginine

34. Green maize is best suited for:

a. Hay making | **b. Silage making**

c. Urea ammoniation | d. Water soaking

35. Higher intake of lush berseem results in to:

a. Constipation | **b. Bloat**

c. Calculi | d. Ataxia]

36. Colour of hay should be:

a. Green | b. Brown

c. Grey | d. Black

37. Vitamin not synthesized in cow:

a. Vitamin A | b. Vitamin B_1

c. Vitamin C | d. Vitamin B_{12}

38. The maximum moisture percent in hay should be:

a. 5 % | b. 10 %

c. 15 % | d. 20 %

39. Vitamin synthesized in the tissues of cattle:

a. Vitamin A & D | b. Vitamin B_1 & B_2

c. Vitamin C & D | d. Vitamin B_{12}

40. The CP content of standard dog diet is:

a. 10 % | b. 15 %

c. 18 % | **d. 22 %**

41. Which is an obligatory carnivorous animal:

a. Dog | b. Monkey

c. Cat | d. Rats

42. The CP content of fresh green maize fodder is:

a. 1.10% | b. 2.50%

c. 3.50% | d. 5.00%

43. The ME content of standard dog diet is:

a. 2 Mcal/kg | b. 3 Mcal/kg

c. 4 Mcal/kg | d. 5 Mcal/kg

44. The CF content of adult rabbit diet should be:

a. 2 %
b. 4 %
c. 8 %
d. 16 %

45. The guinea pig is a:

a. Carnivorous
b. Pig
c. Herbivorous
d. Ruminant

46. Raw egg white injury is caused due to presence of:

a. Biotin
b. Choline
c. Avidine
d. Thiaminase

47. Chelosis is caused due to deficiency of:

a. Vit. B_1
b. Vit. B_2
c. Niacin
d. Vit. B_{12}

48. The efficiency of feed protein utilization for egg production in layers is about:

a. 55 %
b. 64 %
c. 70 %
d. 80 %

49. As per ICAR feeding standard, gestation requirement of DCP for a cow is:

a. 0.14 kg/day
b. 0.30 kg/day
c. 0.54 kg/day
d. 0.70 kg/day

50. In the year 1810, "hay equivalent" feeding standard was proposed by:

a. Grouven
b. Wolff
c. Armsby
d. Thaer

51. Urea-molasses-mineral block is used as a source of:

a. Nitrogen
b. Energy
c. Minerals
d. All of the above

52. The DCP value of wheat straw is:

a. 0 %
b. 4 %
c. 8 %
d. 12 %

53. Copper sulphate is mostly used as a feed additive in the ration of:

a. Cattle **b. Pigs**

c. Buffalo d. Poultry

54. A diet fed to cattle with winder nutritive ratio is an indicative of:

a. Better utilization of feed nutrients

b. Poor utilization of feed nutrients

c. Does not affect the feed nutrient utilization

d. None of the above

55. To calculate TDN, the ether extract (EE) value of feed is multiplied by the factor:

a. 6.25 b. 4.25

c. 2.25 d. 1.41

56. One mole of palmitic acid metabolism in animal body gives a net gain of ATP as:

a. 10 b. 22

c. 38 **d. 129**

57. Which one of the following is associated with deficiency of linoleic acid in guinea pig:

a. Ketosis b. Pica

c. Dermatitis d. Indigestion

58. Glucose is catabolised in anaerobic condition heavy exercise and produces:

a. Acetic cid b. Propionic acid

c. Butyric acid **d. Lactic acid**

59. The most prominent sign of niacin deficiency in pig is:

a. Bloody diarrhoea b. Alopecia

c. Blue tongue d. Skin allergy

60. Feeding of raw egg for prolong time in dog results in deficiency of vitamins:

a. Vitamin-C b. Vitamin-B_2

c. Vitamin-A **d. Biotin**

61. Which one of the following diet is restricted in renal insufficiency:

a. **High protein** b. Low protein

c. Low energy d. Low mineral

62. Microbial protein synthesis occurs in following part of GI tract of horse:

a. Stomach b. Duodenum

c. **Caecum** d. Oesophagus

63. In animal body the reserve of carbohydrate is:

a. Glucose b. **Glycogen**

c. Galactose d. Fructose

64. The quantity of TDN required by a 400 kg cow for maintenance is:

a. 100 gm b. 150 gm

c. **250 gm** d. 300 gm

65. Microbial protein synthesis in the rumen depends upon:

a. Rumen degradable protein

b. Ruminal ammonia concentration

c. ME intake

d. **All of the above**

66. Biological value of rumen microbial protein is:

a. 65 % b. 70 %

c. **80 %** d. 50 %

67. The NRC standards of USA came in to existence in the year:

a. 1935 b. 1975

c. **1945** d. 1930

68. The energy spent in the fasting animal is known:

a. Basal metabolism b. **Fasting catabolism**

c. Heat increment d. Heat of nutrient metabolism

69. The calf should be given colostrum within:

a. 8-12 hrs of birth b. 12-24 hrs of birth

c. 24-36 hrs of birth d. 36-48 hrs of birth

70. The DCP content of an ideal calf starter should be:

a. 14-16 % b. 16-18 %

c. 18-20 % **d. 20-22 %**

71. The best source of phosphorus for cattle is:

a. Wheat straw b. Green maize

c. Wheat bran d. Green berseem

72. The energy requirement of children (3-4 years)/day is:

a. 1000 Kcal b. 1640 Kcal

c. 1240 Kcal d. 1820 Kcal

73. Coprophagy is a common phenomenon in:

a. Dogs b. Pigs

c. Rabbits d. Cats

74. The richest source of beta-carotene is:

a. Drumstick leaves b. Mango fruit

c. Carrot d. Papaya

75. Deficiency of thiamine in human causes:

a. Beri-Beri b. Pellagra

c. Scurvy d. Rickets

76. The BIS specification for crude protein percent in rat's diet is:

a. 40 % b. 10 %

c. 16 % **d. 24 %**

77. The protein (%) in human milk is:

a. 3 b. 3.5

c. 1.2 d. 2.1

78. The fat % in egg-yolk is:

a. 16% b. 18%

c. 32% d. 22%

79. The best source of vitamin E is:

a. Wheat germ oil b. Maize

c. Rice d. Egg

80. TDN is a measure of:

a. Protein **b. Energy**

c. Vitamins d. Minerals

81. Rice polish is:

a. Rich in fat b. Rich in phosphorus

c. Rich in B-complex vitamins **d. All of the above**

82. Molasses are rich source of:

a. Soluble sugars b. Cellulose

c. Proteins d. Vitamins

83. The protein requirement of ruminants according to ARC (1980) is based on:

a. DCP

b. Total crude protein

c. Metabolizable protein

d. Rumen degradable and undegradable protein

84. Colostrum should be fed to new born calf with in:

a. 24 hours b. 48 hours

c. 72 hours d. 96 hours

85. Piglet anaemia occurs due to the deficiency of:

a. Iron b. Manganese

c. Copper d. Zink

86. According to BIS, the CP content in concentrate mixtures of dairy cattle should be:

a. Maximum 16% b. Maximum 16%

c. Minimum 20% d. Maximum 20%

87. With grazing animals, the digestibility coefficients can be calculated indirectly by using:

a. Copper sulphate **b. Chromic oxide**

c. Cobalt bullet d. None of the above is correct

88. Fibre in the diet:

a. Reduces blood glucose concentration

b. Increases bulk and prevents constipation

c. Reduces serum cholesterol

d. All of the above

89. Spices:

a. Are rich in fat

b. Interfere with calcium absorption

c. Are rich in choline and amines

d. Have no antibacterial property

90. Millets are rich in:

a. Soluble carbohydrates b. Phosphorus

c. Vitamin A **d. Tannins**

91. The level of crude fibre in dogs diet varies from:

a. 1-2 % **b. 2.5-5 %**

c. 3.5-7 % d. 7.5-10 %

92. The protein content in the diet of guinea pig should be:

a. 15 % **b. 18 %**

c. 20 % d. 23 %

93. Protein content of commercial cat food is:

a. 10 % b. 20 %

c. 30 % d. 40 %

94. The main source of energy in the diets of poor people in India is:

a. Coarse cereal grains b. Hydrogenated fats

c. Ghee d. Vegetable oils

95. Which of the following diet is relatively more safe and balanced for feeding adult pet dog:

a. Kitchen residue b. Home made foods

c. Milk alone **d. Soft moist commercial diets**

96. NPN stands for:

a. Non nitrogenous protein

b. Non protein nitrogen

c. Normal protein nitrogen

d. None of the above is correct

97. Calf starter should contain:

a. 10% CP **b. 23% CP**

c. 30% CP d. 35% CP

98. Starch equivalent was described by:

a. Thaer b. Hacker

c. Armsby **d. Kellner**

99. Paddy straw:

a. Rich in cellulose b. Do not contain DCP

c. Rich in Oxalates **d. All of the above**

100. Hybrid Napier is a cross between:

a. Bajra and Napier b. Jowar and Napier

c. Jowar and Bajra d. None of the above

101. Addition of antioxidants to rations prevents:

a.	Bloat	b.	Disease occurrence
c.	**Rancidity**	d.	None of the above

102. Milk replacers are introduced into the rations of calves when they attain the age of:

a.	One month	**b.**	**One week**
c.	Two months	d.	Three months

103. Ratio of nitrogen to sulphur for proper wool growth should be:

a.	**10:1**	b.	1:10
c.	12:2	d.	2:12

104. Pulses are rich sources of the following vitamins:

a.	Vitamin A	**b.**	**Vitamin B-complex**
c.	Vitamin C	d.	Vitamin D

105. The protein content in their stock ration contains:

a.	10-12 %	b.	12-14 %
c.	**14-16 %**	d.	16-18 %

106. The requirement of the following vitamin depends upon the caloric intake:

a.	Vitamin A	b.	Vitamin D
c.	**Vitamin B-complex**	d.	Vitamin C

107. The sparing action of selenium on vitamin E is absent in:

a.	**Rabbits**	b.	Cats
c.	Rats	d.	Guinea pigs

108. High cost balanced diets of children mostly consists of:

a.	More quantity of milk	b.	More of meat and eggs
c.	Less of cereals	**d.**	**All of the above**

109. High consumption of the following is contraindicated in pets suffering from diabetes:

a.	Animal proteins	**b.**	**Sugar and starchy feeds**
c.	Green leafy vegetables	d.	Skimmed milk

110. In cardiac insufficiency of dogs:

a. Salt intake should be reduced drastically

b. Fat content of diet should be increased

c. Dietary mineral content should be reduced

d. All of the above

111. The following animal cannot synthesize nicotinic acid from tryptophan:

a. Dog **b. Cat**

c. Rat d. Rabbit

112. Embryonic degeneration in female rat is due to:

a. Vitamin K deficiency b. Vitamin A deficiency

c. Vitamin C deficiency d. Vitamin E deficiency

113. Nutritive value (DCP & TDN) of feedstuff can be determined by:

a. Proximate analysis **b. Digestibility trial**

c. Analysis of fibre fractions d. Feed intake/weight gain

114. In non-ruminant rations:

a. CF can exceed 20 percent

b. Quality of protein is important

c. Urea can be included at 3% level

d. Water soluble vitamins are not essential

115. The energy requirements of ruminants by ARC (1980) are based on:

a. GE b. DE

c. ME d. NE

116. Feed accounted to the cost of production of rabbit is:

a. About 40-50% b. About 50-65%

c. About 70-75% d. About 80-85%

117. Human milk contains:

a. Less protein than animal milk

b. Less casein than animal milk

c. High amount of lactose

d. All of the above

118. Natural indicator (marker) used for determination of digestibility coefficient of feed in animals is:

a.	Chromic oxide	b.	Polyethylene glycol
c.	**Lignin**	d.	Copper sulphate

119. Mice diet is supplemented with:

a.	1.0 % fat	b.	2.0 % fat
c.	**3.0 % fat**	d.	4.0 % fat

120. Normal dry matter intake of dairy cow is:

a.	**2.5 % b.wt.**	b.	1.5 % b.wt.
c.	4.0 % b.wt.	d.	4.5 % b.wt.

121. DCP requirement (g) per kg cow's milk (4% fat) is:

a.	35	**b.**	**45**
c.	65	d.	75

122. One kg of TDN is equal to M cal DE:

a.	3.41	**b.**	**4.41**
c.	5.41	d.	2.41

123. A calf should receive immunoglobulin (gm) during the first 24 hours:

a.	**300-400**	b.	500-600
c.	800-900	d.	1100-1200

124. The protein (%) content of growing pig ration is:

a.	12	b.	13
c.	14	d.	**16**

125. Post absorptive state is achieved when the non-protein R.Q. is :

a.	0.6	**b.**	**0.7**
c.	008	d.	None of the above

126. The ME (Kcal) content to starter chick ration is:

a.	3000	b.	2900
c.	**2800**	d.	2700

127. Milk is deficient in:

a. Biotin b. Vit. B_{12}

c. Iron d. Calcium

128. Pulses are deficient in amino acid:

a. Lysine b. Methionine

c. Tryptophan d. Leucine

129. Which one is not a cereal:

a. Maize b. Oats

c. Barley **d. Gram**

130. The diet for rabbit normally contains dry roughage:

a. 30-40 % **b. 50-70 %**

c. 10-20 % d. 80-90 %

131. Daily recommended allowance of energy (Kcal) for women (45kg body weight) for moderate work is:

a. 2000 **b. 2300**

c. 3300 d. 1800

132. Metabolical energy (Kcal) requirement for a lactating bitch/$W^{0.75}$ kg is:

a. 200 b. 380

c. 470 d. 189

133. Marasmus is a deficiency disease in children due to less intake of:

a. Protein **b. Energy**

c. Mineral d. Vitamins

134. 100 g maize supply protein:

a. 28 g b. 18 g

c. 9 g d. 36 g

135. In which of the following condition nitrogen balance will be positive:

a. Fasting **b. Growth**

c. Prolonged illness d. None of the above

136. The percent amount of every nutrient in any feed which is actually digested in side the body is known as:

a.	Digestion trial	b.	Metabolic trail
c.	**Digestion coefficient**	d.	Digestible energy

137. Pregnancy toxaemia can be prevented by feeding:

a.	Protein rich diet	**b.**	**Energy rich diet**
c.	Vitamin rich diet	d.	Mineral rich diet

138. A complete feed is most economical for fat lamb production with the concentrate: roughage ration:

a.	**50:50**	b.	25:75
c.	75:25	d.	40:60

139. In natural condition goat prefers:

a.	Nibbing	b.	Grazing
c.	**Browsing**	d.	Stall feeding

140. Improving the nutritional status of ewes during 3-4 weeks prior to mating is known as:

a.	Steaming up	**b.**	**Flushing**
c.	Weaning	d.	None of the above

141. For annual production of 4 kg wool, a sheep would require depositing daily:

a.	1.0 g nitrogen	**b.**	**1.3 g nitrogen**
c.	1.6 g nitrogen	d.	1.9 g nitrogen

142. Goat does not relish eating:

a.	Maize fodder	b.	Berseem fodder
c.	Oat fodder	**d.**	**Silage**

143. Valine amino acid is a:

a.	α-amino propionic acid	b.	Amino acetic acid
c.	**α-amino isovaleric acid**	d.	α-amino glutaric acid

144. Amylase is a starch digesting enzyme secreted by the:

a. Gastric gland **b. Pancreas**

c. Intestinal wall d. Caecum

145. Mahuwa flower contains:

a. 40 % TDN **b. 68 % TDN**

c. 50 % TDN d. 85 % TDN

146. Crude fiber is digested in G.I.T. of horse:

a. Stomach b. Duodenum

c. Mouth **d. Caecum**

147. Barley is deficient in vitamin:

a. Vitamin A and D b. Vitamin B and C

c. Vitamin E d. None of the above

148. One international unit of vitamin A is:

a. 0.3 mg vitamin A in alcohol b. 0.4 mg vitamin A in alcohol

c. 0.5 mg vitamin A in alcohol d. 0.6 mg vitamin A in alcohol

149. How many naturally occurring form of vitamin E_1 are there:

a. 2 b. 4

c. 6 **d. 8**

150. The concentrate mixture fed to growing horse may contains:

a. 12-14 % CP b. 15-17 % CP

c. 18-20 % CP d. 21-23 % CP

151. The most economical source of energy of livestock is:

a. Feeds high in fat

b. Feeds high in carbohydrate

c. Feeds high in vitamins

d. Feeds high in proteins

152. Limiting amino acids in poultry diet is:

a. Arginine and histidine

b. Alanine and valine

c. Aspartic acid and glutamic acid

d. Lysine and methionine

153. Dietary essential nutrients are those which are:

a. Found in all animal feeds

b. Provide at the cheaper cost

c. Need for most of the body functions

d. Non-synthesized in adequate amount in relation to their requirements

154. Feeding proteins in excess of animal's requirement:

a. Leads to less excretion of urine

b. Is injurious to kidneys

c. Is not harmful

d. Make them fatty

155. What energy system is recommended by ARC, feeding standards:

a. SE system **b. ME system**

c. NE system d. None of the above

156. DCP requirement for maintenance and last quarter of pregnancy of a cow weighting 400kg:

a. 315 g b. 240 g

c. 290 g **d. 355 g**

157. TDN requirement of a bullock weighting 500 kg for normal work:

a. 3.2 kg b. 4.0 kg

c. 4.9 kg d. 6.2 kg

158. ME Kcal/kg diet of growing chicks (0-6 weeks):

a. 2500 b. 3400

c. 2900 d. 4300

159. In practice common salt is generally added to the diet of laboratory animals at a level of :

a. 1.0 % b. 2.0 %

c. 0.5 % d. 0.25 %

160. Percent protein in the diet of lactating does is :

a. 12 b. 22

c. 30 d. 10

161. Percent calcium in the diet of bunnies is :

a. 0.2 **b. 0.4**

c. 0.8 d. 1.0

162. Conversion of GE in feed of poultry into human food (eggs):

a. 7 % b. 15 %

c. 10 % d. 20 %

163. The energy in Indian diet is supplied by the carbohydrates and fat approximately :

a. 50 % b. 70 %

c. 90 % d. 100 %

164. Spinach is a rich source of :

a. Vitamin B_{12} b. Calcium

c. Phosphorus **d. Iron**

165. Percent protein in wheat flour is :

a. 1.6 b. 6.0

c. 10.6 d. 20.1

166. Raw soyabean contain an antinutritioanl factor is :

a. Gossypol b. Nitrate

c. Aflatoxin **d. Trypsin inhibitor**

167. Digestion of feed nutrients results in:

a. Absorption into blood

b. Utilization by the animal body

c. Conversion of soluble compounds

d. Conversion of insoluble compounds

168. Armsby feeding standards is based on:

a. SE system b. ME system

c. NE system d. None of the above

169. Percent CF in a creep ration is:

a. Less than 5 b. Less than 15

c. More than 20 d. More than 30

170. TDN requirement of sheep for maintenance (25kg BW):

a. 250 g **b. 350 g**

c. 450 g d. 550 g

171. DCP requirement for maintenance of Indian cows weighting 400 kg is:

a. 240-250 g b. 260-300 g

c. 300-400 g d. 210-220 g

172. Caloric/protein ratio in the diet of broiler finisher (6-9 weeks):

a. 140:1 **b. 160:1**

c. 110:1 d. 190:1

173. Total nitrogen intake of adult ruminants can be safely replaced by urea nitrogen:

a. 100 % b. 80 %

c. 60 % **d. 30 %**

174. Concentrate mixture for rabbit feeding contains on an average:

a. 40 % TDN **b. 60 % TDN**

c. 80 % TDN d. 20 % TDN

175. Conversion of GE in the feed of pigs into human food (pork):

a. 10 % **b. 20 %**

c. 30 % d. 50 %

176. Percent protein in the diet of guinea pigs:

a. 10 **b. 20**

c. 30 d. 50

177. Daily recommend allowance of vitamin A for adolescent boy and girls:

a. 1000-2000 IU b. 2000-3000 IU

c. 3000-4000 IU d. 4000-5000 IU

178. 100 g rice supply protein:

a. 28 g **b. 7 g**

c. 15 g d. 2 g

179. Who identified essential amino acids for animals and human:

a. W.O.Twater **b. W.C.Rose**

c. W.J.Miller d. W.S.Harr

180. Copper sulphate and zinc oxide are added in per ton of mineral mixture:

a. 22 gm and 11 gm b. 30 gm and 15 gm

c. 40 gm and 20 gm d. 50 gm and 25 gm

181. Antibiotics are added in creep ration of goat:

a. To check pathogenic organism

b. As a growth promotor

c. To check the growth of fungus

d. To control parasitic disease

182. The nutrient conversion efficiency in goat range from:

a. 20-40% **b. 40-60%**

c. 60-80% d. 80-100%

183. The inhibition of methane production in rumen could be:

a. Disadvantageous **b. Advantageous**

c. Decreased feed efficiency d. None of these

184. pKa values of volatile fatty acid are :

a. 3.75-3.30 **b. 4.75-4.80**

c. 5.75-5.80 d. 6.75-6.80

185. For every litres of milk produced the water needed by the cow is:

a. 1.0-1.5 b. 2.0-2.5

c. 3.0-3.5 d. 4.0-4.5

186. Degnala is the disease of:

a. Bacteria | b. Fungus

c. Toxicity of selenium | d. Toxicity of molybdenum

187. Feed stuffs containing more than 18% crude fibre is called:

a. Concentrate | **b. Roughage**

c. Feed supplement | d. Feed additive

188. DCP requirement for guinea pig is:

a. 18 % | **b. 22 %**

c. 24 % | d. 26 %

Q.3. Fill in the blanks :

1. Pigs can digest crude fiber to some extent and fiber digestion is entirely dependent upon bacterial fermentation in ***caecum and colon.***
2. Paralysis of legs due to deficiency of vitamin B_2 (riboflavin) in poultry is termed as ***curled toe paralysis.***
3. Polyneuritis in poultry is caused due to deficiency of vitamin ***B_1 or thiamine.***
4. Wool is a protein which is especially rich in amino acid ***cystine.***
5. A disease specific is ducks marked by bowed leg condition is caused due to deficiency of ***niacin.***
6. The general recommendation for feeding colostrum to calves is ***one tenth*** of body weight.
7. Feeding of some quantity of animal source of proteins to poultry is recommended because animal source of proteins are rich in ***essential amino acids.***
8. A syndrome consisting of alopecia, dermatitis and loss of crimp in wool is due to deficiency of ***copper.***
9. The crude protein requirement of cat is significantly higher than dogs and is about ***34%*** of the diet.
10. The separation of fiber and non-fiber component in hind gut of rabbit takes place at ***caeco-colic*** junction.
11. The phenomenon of consuming its faeces directly from the anus in rabbits is called ***coprophagy.***

12. Contrary to ruminants where propionic acid is second highest volatile fatty acid in rumen, ***butyric acid*** is the second highest volatile fatty acid in the caecum of rabbits.

13. A severe protein energy deficiency manifested by extreme waisting of muscles and other tissues, hair changes and irritability in children is called ***marasmus.***

14. The body building foodstuffs contain a satisfactory amount of nutrients needed to build the body and replace worn out tissues are generally rich in ***protein.***

15. A disease characterized by swelling of thyroid gland in the neck and resulting from deficiency of iodine is called ***goiter.***

16. The daily energy requirement recommended by ICMR for an adult man performing heavy work is ***3900*** kcal/day.

17. Formula for calculating N.E. for maintenance of cow= $80W^{0.75}$.

18. For 500 kg lactating cow, DCP requirement for maintenance is ***300 g.***

19. In a metabolism trial ***urine*** is also collected along with faeces.

20. Quantity of E.U.N. excreted per kg metabolic body size is ***146 mg.***

21. Broiler starters require ***23%*** C.P. in ration.

22. Colostrum contains ***5*** times more protein than normal milk in cows.

23. Fresh green barseem contains ***2.5%*** D.C.P.

24. Fish meal should contain>***60%*** C.P.

25. The protein content of pulse is between ***18-24 percent.***

26. Groundnut contains about ***20%*** protein and ***45%*** fat.

27. Soybean contains about ***45%*** protein and ***20%*** fat.

28. Cats have higher dietary requirement of ***fats*** and ***protein*** than dogs.

29. National Research Council (NRC) published nutrient requirements for livestock for the first time during the year ***1945.***

30. Water soaking of paddy straw removes ***soluble oxalate*** otherwise it affects mineral metabolism in animals.

31. In Beckmann process of straw treatment, the material is treated with ***NaOH*** chemical.
32. The CP content of sugarcane molasses is ***3-4%.***
33. *Mahua* seed contains anti-nutritional factor known as ***mawrine (saponin).***
34. The mimosine present in subabul is degraded to ***2-4 dihydroxy pyridine*** in the rumen of cattle.
35. The TDN requirement for maintenance in adult goat is ***30g/kgW$^{0.75}$***
36. Supplementation of phenylalanine in the diet of pig fulfills the requirement of ***tyrosine*** amino acid.
37. The enzyme responsible for the conversion of glucose to vitamin C is ***L-gluconolactone dehydrogenase.***
38. The recommended allowances of fiber in dog diet are ***5-10%*** on DM basis.
39. Corn oil is rich in essential fatty acid ***linoleic acid.***
40. Dogs are not able to digest raw starch due to the absence of ***amylase*** enzyme.
41. One gram of fat produces ***1 to 1.07*** ml of metabolic water.
42. The most popular grain used in horse feeding ***oats.***
43. Cats are very sensitive to the deficiency of ***arginine*** amino acid.
44. The amino acid tryptophan may be converted to ***niacin*** vitamin in animal body.
45. An ideal calf starter should contain ***20-23%*** DCP and ***70%*** TDN
46. ARC feeding standard of UK is based on the ***net energy*** system.
47. The protein content of colostrum is about ***17 percent.***
48. Crude fibre in pig ration should not be more than ***10 percent.***
49. Dry milk replacer powder is mixed in boiled water in the ratio of ***1:4 to 1:5.***
50. Normally about ***70 %*** dry matter should be from roughage in dairy animals.

51. The maintenance requirement of a 400 kg cow is ***0.224*** kg DCP and ***3.5*** kg TDN.
52. In mature dairy animals, urea can replace satisfactorily up to about ***30-40***% of the dietary protein.
53. Body is composed of ***96%*** organic and ***4%*** inorganic elements.
54. ***Safflower*** oil is the richest source of polyunsaturated fatty acids.
55. Richest source of carotene is ***coriander leaves.***
56. ***Vitamin E*** is a natural antioxidant.
57. ***Glucose*** is indispensable for nervous system.
58. ***Vitamin A*** is an anti infective vitamin.
59. ***Poly unsaturated fatty acid*** acts as precursor of prostaglandins.
60. ***Carbohydrates*** are not dietary essential in case of dogs.
61. Average daily ME requirement of growing Pig is ***3250*** Kcal/kg diet.
62. Maximum crude fibre content in the poultry ration should be ***6-8%.***
63. The requirement of crude protein for an adult pig is ***13%*** of the ration.
64. Parakeratosis in the pigs is caused due to the deficiency of ***zinc.***
65. The first limiting amino acid in GNC is ***methionine.***
66. Deficiency of ***riboflavin*** in poultry causes curled toe paralysis.
67. Pica in cattle is due to the deficiency of ***phosphorus.***
68. On an all roughage ration the predominant VFA produced in the rumen is ***acetic acid.***
69. Average daily ME requirement of actively growing 10kg GSD dog is ***1540 Kcal.***
70. The maximum CF content in the rabbit diet should be ***15 percent.***
71. As per BIS (1992), the broiler starter ration should contain ***23%*** crude protein.
72. NRC stands for ***national research council.***
73. One gram of TDN is equivalent to ***4.4*** Kcal of DE.

74. Fibre in adult swine rations should not exceed ***8 percent.***

75. The energy requirements of ARC (1980) for ruminants are based on ***metabolizable*** energy system.

76. Cotton seed meal contains ***gossypol*** as a toxic factor.

77. A byproduct rich in cellulose derived from sugar cane industry is ***bagasse.***

78. Top feeds are rich in ***tannins*** which hinders protein utilization.

79. Pulses are rich in ***protein*** while cereals are rich in ***starch.***

80. The availability of calcium from green leafy vegetables is lowered due to the presence of ***oxalates.***

81. In human beings, carbohydrates are stored as ***glycogen.***

82. Excessive heating may lead to ***browing/mailard*** reaction affecting the availability of amino acids.

83. An expansion of RDA is ***recommended daily allowance.***

84. Raw egg contains ***avidin*** as antivitamin.

85. As per BIS, layer mash should contain ***17%*** crude protein.

86. One kg of TDN is equivalent to ***3.61*** Mcal ME.

87. The finisher diet of swine should contain ***16%*** crude protein.

88. Utilization of unconventional feeds livestock feeding is restricted due to the presence of ***toxic/antinutritional*** factors.

89. Sen and Ray feeding standards are based on ***Morrison's*** feeding standards.

90. Maize is used as a source of ***energy*** while formulating broiler diets.

91. F.C.M. stands for ***fat corrected milk.***

92. The maximum permissible level of crude fibre in the concentrate mixtures of dairy cattle as per BIS is ***12-13 %.***

93. Colostrum contains ***17%*** protein.

94. Highly polished rice consumption leads to the deficiency of ***vitamin*** B_1***/ thiamine*** B-complex vitamin.

95. Among essential fatty acids, arachidonic acid cannot be synthesized from ***linolcic acid*** in all laboratory animals, except cat.

96. Absence of fat in the diet of human beings leads to a condition known as ***phrynoderma.***

97. Rats suffer from acrodynia due to the deficiency of ***vitamin B_6/pyridoxine*** B-complex vitamin.

98. The rich source of iron in Indian vegetarian diets is ***green leafy vegetables.***

99. ***Protein*** foods are contra indicated during renal failure in dogs and cat.

100. Colostrum is rich in ***globulin*** which helps in immunity.

101. ***200 g*** DCP and ***2.4 kg*** TDN are required to meet daily maintenance requirements of 300 kg mature cow.

102. As per BIS, the calorie-protein ratio in starter and laying chicken feeds should be ***122*** and ***144*** respectively.

103. The DMI of dairy goats range from ***4 to 6%*** of their body weight.

104. The CF in adult swine ration should not exceed ***8 percent.***

105. Breeding rams should be provided with ***50%*** more nutrients than the maintenance needs.

106. As per NRC (1994), breeding duck ration should contain ***15%*** protein and ***2900*** Kcal ME/kg diet.

107. ***45*** g DCP and ***0.315*** kg TDN is required for the production of 1kg 4% FCM in cows.

108. Canned dog food normally contains ***75%*** moisture.

109. Sparing action of selenium on vitamin E is absent in ***rabbit.***

110. ***Cat*** (animal) cannot synthesize nicotinic acid from tryptophan.

111. High consumption of ***sugar/starchy*** rich feeds are contraindicated in pets suffering from diabetes.

112. Dogs and cats do not require a dietary supply of ***vit.C/ascorbic acid*** (vitamin) because of its synthesis from glucose.

113. ***Atherosclerosis*** condition results due to an excess deposition of fat cholesterol under the lining of blood vessels.

114. Wolf feeding standard is based on ***digestibility*** of feedstuffs.

115. Crude fiber content in broiler diet should not be more than ***6 percent.***

116. After weaning ***iron*** deficiency is not a serious problem in pigs.
117. BMR (Kcal/d) in adult animals can be calculated by using formula ***$70W^{0.75}$Kg***.
118. Urea can be included @ ***1%*** in the total feed.
119. ***Mimosine*** is a toxic substance present in subabool.
120. The grinding of roughage ***decreases*** the digestibility of dry matter.
121. Sheep grazing on pasture consume ***10%*** more DM than stall fed.
122. ***Methionine*** is the first limiting amino acid in canines.
123. The heat treatment of food by scalding and parboiling in water or steam prior to freezing or canning is known as ***seasoning.***
124. The most common mineral supplement used in human diet is ***zinc.***
125. Rabbits generally prefer ***pellet*** diet than mash.
126. ***Egg*** is a food of animal origin and is very rich in amino acid lysine.
127. Rabbit do not require vitamin B_{12} because of ***coprophagy.***
128. Dogs and cats are ***carnivorous*** animals.
129. Goats are having ***mobile*** lips.
130. Feeding high concentrate in the ration of milch animals cause ***depression in milk fat.***
131. Site of urea formation in the body is ***liver.***
132. Biological value of protein for ruminant is ***70 percent.***
133. DM water intake ratio in goat is ***1:4.***
134. 3 g SE/g live weight gain is required as energy for ***growing*** kid.
135. The capacity of rumen of adult goat is ***28 litres.***
136. The limiting factors present in tree leaves are ***tannins.***
137. Full form of BIS is ***Bureau of Indian standards.***
138. Fructose contains ***Co.***
139. Trehlose sugar is found in ***fungi.***
140. Cephalin is a ***phosphatidyl choline.***

141. Amount of Co_2 produced in the caecum of horse is ***40 to 50 percent.***

142. Acetylation of fatty acid requires ***acetic anhydrase.***

143. Arachidonic acid is an ***essential fatty acid.***

144. Digestibility expressed in percentage is known as ***digestibility coefficient.***

145. A marker ***chromic oxide*** commonly used for determining the digestibility in pigs.

146. A balanced concentrate mixture is prepared in such a manner so that 3.5 to 4.0 kg may support ***10kg*** milk production in cows.

147. A bullock is usually fed at the rate of ***2.5*** kg DM/100kg body weight.

148. Not more than ***one*** percent urea of the total DM intake generally fed to cattle.

149. ***Three*** sets of digestibility traits are conducted to determine the digestibility of non maintenance type of roughages such as straw.

150. Feeding of antibiotics ***increases*** the efficiency of feed utilization in poultry.

151. Calves are fed whole milk at the rate of ***one tenth*** of body weight for first to three weeks of age for optimum growth.

152. Cercal grains for human consumption are generally deficient in essential amino acid ***lysine.***

153. Green vegetables are ***low*** in calorie.

154. Growing children require the entire ***10*** essential amino acid in the diet.

155. Protein requirement for adult man is usually ***1g*** per kg body weight per day.

156. Birth weight of a child becomes ***double*** in 6months of age.

157. Blood cholesterol level increases when it contains more ***saturated*** fatty acids.

158. The BMR is ***higher*** in infant than in adult person.

159. A food of animal source rich in sulphur containing amino acid is ***egg.***

160. Wheat bran is a rich source of mineral ***phosphorus.***

161. Tree leaves contain ***tannins*** which ***decrease*** the digestibility of nutrients.

162. Energy requirement for maintenance can be determined by ***C-N balance*** studies.

163. Diet containing ***2.8*** Mcal energy per kg and ***16 percent*** protein is adequate for laying hen.

164. Zebu cattle have ***lower BMR*** than exotic cattle.

165. A lactating buffalo requires ***more*** energy than a lactating cow.

166. The ideal concentrate mixture should contain ***15-16*** percent DCP and ***70-75*** percent TDN.

167. The chaffing of roughages improves the nutritive value by increasing the ***surface area*** for the microbial action.

168. Purified milk protein is known as ***casein.***

169. Adult human body contains ***63*** percent water.

170. A food of animal's origin very rich in amino acid lysine is ***fish.***

171. Glycolipid contains sugar ***galactose.***

172. Rabbits excrete two types of faecal matter ***hard and soft.***

173. Leafy vegetables are rich source of iron and ***carotene.***

174. A substance used in making bread is very rich in vitamin B-complex ***yeast.***

175. Milk generally contains significant amount of all the essential minerals except ***iron.***

176. Niacin deficiency causes ***pellagra*** in human beings.

177. Steaming up process lead to production of ***healthy*** lamb.

178. Biological value of milk ***replacer*** is equivalent to milk.

179. Feeding extra concentrate mixture to most heavy demand unborn lamb is known as ***steaming up.***

180. Improving the nutritional status of ewes during 3-4 weeks prior to mating is known as ***flushing up.***

181. ***Muscular dystrophy*** is caused by vitamin E deficiency in lamb.

182. Oil cake having maximum crude protein is ***ground nut cake.***

183. Lignin is classified under ***carbohydrate.***

184. Indian cattle maintain body temperature through ***dewlap.***
185. Cryptoxanthine is a provitamin of ***vitamin A.***
186. Mycoxanthine is derived from ***blue green algae.***
187. Poor quality wool productions in rabbit occur in the deficiency of ***sulphur.***
188. Salt sickness occurs in the deficiency of ***copper.***
189. Water requirement of doe rabbit is ***0.6 litres per kg.***
190. ***Parathyroid*** hormone regulates calcium level in plasma.
191. Erepsin is an enzyme secreted from the wall of ***small intestine.***
192. Fats are digested in ***alkaline*** medium only.

8

Livestock Producton & Management (Part-I) Fodder Production and Grassland Management, Animal Husbandry and Sanitation

Q.1. True or False :

1.	True	The body colour of Beetal goat is jet black.
2.	True	Jaisalmeri breed of camel is famous for riding.
3.	True	Pica disease in animals is caused due to the deficiency of phosphorus.
4.	True	Jersey is an exotic breed of cattle.
5.	False	Shearing in sheep is done in the month of December.
6.	False	In India, goats are primarily reared for milk production.
7.	True	Indian cattle maintain body temperature through dewlap.
8.	False	Heavier animals require less water.
9.	True	Zebu cattle require less water than exotic breed.
10.	False	In loose house, 20-25 percent more animals can be accommodated for shorter period.
11.	False	Sorghum is a rabi season non leguminous fodder.
12.	False	FOS-I is a variety of guar.
13.	True	FS-277 variety of cowpea is an erect growing variety.

14. False For hay making crop should be harvested when it is in full bloom stage.

15. True Maize can be harvested 40-45 days after sowing.

16. True Single cut crops should be harvested at 70 percent flowering stage.

17. True Bajra is grown as dual purpose crop.

18. True Sty is the housing place for pigs.

19. False Lambing is the act of parturition in goats.

20. False Raised hair coat is the sign of good health.

21. False Colostrum provides active immunity to the newly born calf.

22. True A teaser bull is maintained to detect heat in cows.

23. True Montgomery is the place of origin of Sahiwal breed.

24. False Special feeding during advanced stage of pregnancy is called flushing.

25. False Foaling is the act of parturition in sheep.

26. True Feeding of green fodder is essential for higher milk production.

27. True Nutritive value of fodder is improved by mixed cropping of cereals and legumes.

28. True Maize is also a good fodder crop in winter season.

29. False Seed treatment with rhizobium culture is associated with sorghum.

30. False Seed rate of lucerne is 12 kg/acre.

31. False HCN poisoning is associated with pearl millet fodder.

32. True Sugar cane tops are fed as scarcity fodder.

33. True The best stage of harvesting cowpea is when 10-15 percent plants have seed pod formation.

34. True The orientation of dairy buildings should be in the east-west direction.

35. True Heat detection is efficient in loose housing system.

36. True Temporary hardness of water is due to the presence of sulphate of calcium and magnesium.

37. False Pond water is good for drinking of dairy animals.

38. True Permanent hardness of water cannot be removed by simple boiling.

39. False Roof of animal houses should be a good conductor of heat.

40. True Water of deep tube well is wholesome.

41. True Lime powder is a common disinfectant at dairy farm.

42. False Chokla is a sheep breed from eastern Kerala.

43. False Tharparkar cattle are roan in colour.

44. False Kathiawari horse breed is from West Bengal.

45. True Sheep/goats become full mouth at around 4 to 4.5 years of age.

46. False Dehorning of goats is done on all organized farms.

47. False Quarantine is not needed for the animals transported from other countries to India.

48. True Daily intake of water in adult sheep is around 4 to 5 litre.

49. False Under field conditions, A.I. is most common in pigs.

50. False Barseem is a non-leguminous fodder crop.

51. False Oat is fed to animals during winter season.

52. True Cow pea is leguminous in nature.

53. True Ranch system of animal production is common in western countries.

54. False Silage is made during period of fodder scarcity.

55. False Horse is ruminant in nature.

56. False Jwar is a leguminous crop.

57. False Silage is stored in open air.

58. True Animal houses should be made up of locally available cheaper material in spite of costlier ones.

59. False Indian climate requires similar type of housing in different agro-climatic zones of our country.

60. False There is no need to construct sheds as per the specified floor requirements for different categories of animals.

61. False — Cattle/buffalo sheds need barbed wire fencing.

62. False — Cement concrete roofing is always recommended for construction of animal sheds.

63. False — An animal farm does not require organized drainage system.

64. True — The genetic ability of an animal breed to cope with higher temperature extremes is generally termed as heat tolerance.

65. True — Incidence of mastitis is influenced by the type of housing system.

66. True — Camel is not a true ruminant animal.

67. False — Brushing the body of animals makes their hair coat hard.

68. False — Surti buffalo has curled shape horns.

69. True — In summers the water intake of animal increases to 10 percent in spite of decline in feed intake.

70. False — The size and number of manure pits depends on the area of the farm.

71. True — Ventilation helps in removing bad odour from the houses.

72. False — For maximum exposure to sun, the dairy barns must have a long exit on the east-west direction.

73. True — Ventilation in animal house by doors is a valuable means of ventilation but not reliable and permanent.

74. True — The effectiveness of ventilation by openings in the walls depends on wind velocity.

75. False — Sunlight admitted through ventilation must produce glare in the house.

76. False — Barseem is the best fodder for silage making.

77. False — Straw is better than hay.

78. True — Guar is a common green fodder fed in rainfed areas.

79. False — Leguminous fodders are rich in carbohydrates.

80. True — Barseem is a leguminous fodder.

81. False — In hay making loss of dry matter due to leaves is 5 to 20 percent.

82.	True	The act of mating in sheep is called tupping.
83.	False	Falling of animal on the ground is known as restraining.
84.	False	The pigs of Large White Yorkshire breed have freckles and loopy ears.
85.	True	White leghorn is the best egg producing strain.
86.	True	Hariana is a dual purpose breed of cattle.
87.	False	There are four incisors in the upper jaw of cattle.
88.	True	Best age of castration of male Zebu cattle is 12 to15 months.
89.	True	The hybrid Napier grass is a perennial fodder crop.
90.	False	Roughages contain less than 15 percent crude fibre.
91.	True	Lucerne is best for hay making.
92.	True	The appropriate stage of harvesting oat fodder crop is dough stage.
93.	True	In hot humid regions fodder grows faster and lignified earlier.
94.	False	Urea fertilizer is a good source of both nitrogen and phosphorus.
95.	False	Feeding of maize fodder in summer leads to HCN toxicity in animals.
96.	True	Indian pastures/grazing lands are seriously lacking in legume grasses.
97.	False	There is efficient heat detection in CB system of housing.
98.	True	The river water is dangerous for drinking of animals.
99.	True	The inlet is used for expiration of foul air from barn.
100.	True	The adverse effect of high temperature is more if accompanied with high humidity.
101.	False	Disease control is always easier in loose housing system.
102.	True	There is a negative correlation between milk yield and ambient temperature.
103.	True	The CB system is suitable under temperate climatic conditions.

104.	True	The temperature humidity index (THI) helps in decision-making on ventilation.
105.	True	The act of birth in case of pigs is called farrowing.
106.	False	White Cornish breed of chicken belong to the American class.
107.	False	The pigs of Landrace breed have six white spots on the body.
108.	False	The gestation period in case of sheep is 112-114 days.
109.	True	The popular name of Nili-Ravi buffalo is Panch Phooli or Panch Kalyani.
110.	True	Kankrej bullocks are famous for swai-chal.
111.	True	The best method of milking cow is fisting.
112.	False	Mule is a hybrid of Jannet and horse stallion.
113.	False	Lucerne is the best fodder for silage milking.
114.	True	Phosphate fertilizers are required for barseem crops.
115.	False	Hay is the succulent fermented and preserved fodder.
116.	False	Good quality hay is prepared from thick-stem, ripened fodder cross.
117.	True	Feeding of sorghum in dough stage lead to HCN toxicity.
118.	True	The stocking density is more than 30 times of carrying capacity of grazing lands in India.
119.	False	Maize is the best fodder for hay making.
120.	True	The thermal neutral zone (TNZ) varies from species to species.
121.	False	The covered area provided to a cow is 4 square meter in LH system.
122.	False	The relative humidity in loose housing system is always more as compared to CB system.
123.	True	Low heat liberation in shed is achieved by low stocking density.
124.	True	Kings Ventilation method is used in cold climatic conditions.
125.	False	Disease control is difficult in CB system.

126. True The device used to check back flow in a drainage system is called trap.

127. True Barbari goats are commonly found in Agra area of U.P.

128. False Angora goats are reared for pashmina production.

129. False Jaffarabadi buffalo's milk has got highest fat content among all buffalo breeds.

130. False Ankamali is a chinese pig breed.

131. False The population of Kathiawadi horses has increased during last 50 years.

132. False The native place of Karaknath breed of poultry is in Assam.

133. True Mithun is not reared for milk production.

134. False Brick walls are cheap and common for animal house construction in hills.

135. False Slatted floors are most common for buffaloes.

136. False The cement concrete floor is most comfortable and common for sheep.

137. False Paddy straw is best thatching material for livestock housing.

138. True Mercury is a non-degradable pollutant.

139. True Nitrate water pollution is the result of improper use of fertilizers in crops.

140. True Breeding seasonality in livestock is related to photoperiodism.

141. False The wind velocity reduces the ventilation in natural condition.

142. False Sandy soil is best suited for barseem cultivation.

143. False Leguminous crops need higher nitrogen supplementation.

144. False Clovers are best suited for silage making.

145. True Cowpea can be cultivated as mixed crop with maize.

146. True Cultivation of leguminous and non leguminous crop alternatively is good for soil health.

147. False The traditional varieties of sorghum should be cultivated during hot and dry season.

148. False — Soil pH should be 8.0 for good fodder cultivation.

149. False — Oat is a perennial crop.

150. True — Animals of Holstein Friesian breed are the best milk producers in the world.

151. True — Murrah buffalo breed is most popular especially in northern India.

152. False — Hariana breed of cattle is a draught purpose breed.

153. True — Jersey, an exotic breed of cattle is considered to be more suitable for hilly areas.

154. False — Cows of Sahiwal breed produce less milk as compared to other indigenous breeds.

155. False — GIR is the draught cattle breed of India.

156. True — Tharparkar is not a good dual purpose breed of cattle.

157. False — Pure air is found in the immediate vicinity of animals or people.

158. True — Free ammonia resulting from decomposition of urea is found in the air of badly constructed and badly ventilated animal houses.

159. True — The most extreme instance of heat resulting from badly ventilated buildings is seen in heat stroke which may cause death of the animal.

160. True — All young animals should have an access to adequate amount of direct sunlight.

161. False — In laying hens, egg production cannot be influenced considerably by the amount of light to which the birds are subjected.

162. False — Direct sunlight has no germicidal action.

163. True — Tubercle bacilli when spread in a thin layer are not destroyed in few hours if exposed to the direct rays of sun.

164. True — As an aid to better lighting and cleanliness, the upper part of the walls and the ceiling in animal building should be white.

165. True — Fodder and grazing resources of India have become inadequate to meet the needs of the livestock population.

166. True — Grazing and fodder resources contribute to greater efficiency from the working animals.

167. True — Dairy animals require highest available form of fodder production with continuous supply of high quality green and other feeds throughout the year.

168. False — India is a year round grazing country.

169. False — In India, during effective grazing season, the nutritive value of the herbage at its best is such that it can always provide both a maintenance and production ration for high quality livestock.

170. True — Fodder species are available for inclusion in the farming system in most part of India.

171. False — Fodder species represent a very large percentage of total area under cultivated crops.

172. False — Cereal straws (BHUSA), JUAR stalks (KADBI) and other crop residues do not provide the main fodder in India.

173. True — Jamunapari breed of goat is found in Etawah.

174. True — Chevon is the name given to meat of goat.

175. True — Mohair is obtained from Angora goats.

176. True — Kankrej breed of cow is the heaviest and most powerful.

177. False — Red Dane is a breed of buffalo.

178. False — Jersey is not an exotic breed of cow.

179. True — Tharparkar is a dual purpose breed of cow.

180. False — Mutton is the name given to meat of poultry.

181. False — In India the total cultivated area under fodder crop is more than 10 percent.

182. True — Lucerne crop of fodder is a perennial crop.

183. True — *Lasirus sindicus* is the botanical name of sewan.

184. False — Hybrid Napier is a single cut fodder crop.

185. False — Feed materials can safely be stored at high moisture and very low temperature.

186. False — The variable cost does not affect the cost of fodder and milk production.

187. True — Yellow colour in cow's milk occurs due to carotene.

188. False — Under loose housing system, the covered area required per cattle is 100 square feet.

189. True — Outlet ventilators should not be fixed at about 2 feet height.

190. True — Plumbism is due to poisoning of lead.

191. True — Degree of hardness of moderately hard water is less than 3-6.

192. True — In summer exhaust fans should be placed high in cattle sheds.

193. False — Space requirement per broiler at 5 weeks age is 2 square feet.

Q.2. Multiple Choice Questions :

1. The colour of Holstein Friesian breed is:

   a. Fawn **b. Black and White**

   c. Reddish d. Grey

2. Washing of teats is done:

   a. To increase milk production

   b. To stimulate let down of milk

   c. For quick milking

   d. To get more fat in milk

3. Camel belongs to the family:

   a. Equidae b. Bovidae

   c. Suidae **d. Camelidae**

4. The disease where carcass must be pitted with lime:

   a. Anthrax b. Black quarter

   c. Tuberculosis d. Malaria

5. Which one of the following is a disinfectant:

   a. Chloroform **b. Chlorine**

   c. Potassium nitrate d. Boric acid

6. White leghorn fowl belongs to:

   a. American class
   b. Asiatic class
   c. English class
   d. Mediterranean class

7. After birth umbilical cord must be treated with:

   a. Sodium carbonate
   b. Potassium permanganate
   c. Sulphur ointment
   d. Tincture iodine

8. Mark the lyre horned grey cattle with wide forehead and flat or dished in profile:

   a. Hariana
   b. Sahiwal
   c. Amritmahal
   d. Kankrej

9. Thickness of concrete walls should be:

   a. 10 cm
   b. 12 cm
   c. 15 cm
   d. 18 cm

10. Most suitable place for inlet of fresh air in animal house is:

    a. Top of the house
    b. At the floor level
    c. Top of the manger
    d. None of the above

11. The best advantage of round barn is:

    a. Low cost
    b. Even distribution of light
    c. Centrally located silo
    d. Easy cleaning of gutter

12. Maximum number of buffaloes that can be kept per pen:

    a. 30
    b. 40
    c. 60
    d. 50

13. Floor space requirement for older calves under covered area is:

    a. 3.0 m^2
    b. 2.0 m^2
    c. 2.5 m^2
    d. 1.0 m^2

14. Ideal ambient temperature range of adaptation for exotic breed:

    a. 5-10^{0}C
    b. 0-16^{0}C
    c. 10-20^{0}C
    d. 10-15^{0}C

15. Width of farm gates towards road should be:

    a. 2.0 metres **b. 2.5 metres**

    c. 1.5 metres d. 3.0 metres

16. FOS-1 is a variety of:

    a. Barseem b. **Cowpea**

    c. Lucerne d. Guar

17. Name the scarcity fodder:

    a. Maize b. Bajra

    c. Sugarcane top d. Sorghum

18. Name the leguminous fodder:

    a. Sugarcane tops **b. Barseem**

    c. Maize d. Hybrid Napier

19. Carotene losses in field curing method per kg is:

    a. 10 mg b. 7 mg

    c. 12 mg d. 14 mg

20. Best crop for silage making in rabi season is:

    a. Barseem **b. Oat**

    c. Lucerne d. Barley

21. Which crop is used as a green fodder:

    a. Moong b. Wheat

    c. Sorghum d. Barley

22. Succulent fermented preserved green fodder is known as:

    a. Hay b. Herbage

    c. Silage d. Forage

23. At the time of silage making crop should contain dry matter:

    a. 30-40 percent **b. 25-30 percent**

    c. 20-25 percent d. 15-20 percent

24. Mark the oestrus cycle of a healthy cow:

a. 15 days **b. 21 days**

c. 28 days d. None of the above

25. A vasectomised male cattle can be used as:

a. Teaser b. Bull

c. Steer d. None of the above

26. The best method of hand milking in cows is:

a. Dry & full hand b. Wet hand

c. Knuckling d. None of the above

27. The buffalo breed which has jet black colour and tightly curved horns:

a. Bhadawari **b. Murrah**

c. Surti d. None of the above

28. The gestation period of cow is:

a. 151 days **b. 282 days**

c. 340 days d. None of the above

29. Holding up of milk in cow is due to the effect of:

a. Adrenaline b. Oxytocin

c. Progesterone d. None of the above

30. After birth calf should be fed colostrum:

a. Within ½ - 2 hours b. After 6-8 hours

c. After discharge of placenta d. None of the above

31. Mark the ideal pH of good silage:

a. 2.2 – 3.5 **b. 4.2 – 4.5**

c. 5.2 – 5.5 d. None of the above

32. Seed rate of barseem fodder per acre is:

a. 5 – 6 mg **b. 9 – 10 kg**

c. 15-16 kg d. None of the above

33. How many buffaloes can be maintained on one acre fodder land:

a. 3 **b. 5**

c. 10 d. None of the above

34. In per cubic feet area of silo pit how much of the silage can be stored:

a. 8-10 kg **b. 15-16 kg**

c. 25-26 kg. d. None of the above

35. Mark the number of root/stem cuttings required for sowing one acre of napier grass:

a. 5000 **b. 11000**

c. 16000 d. None of the above

36. One ACU is equal to how many adult sheep and goats:

a. 5 b. 10

c. 15 d. None of the above

37. The best fodder crop for hay making is:

a. Lucerne b. Maize

c. Teosinte d. None of the above

38. Maximum number of cows kept in a dairy shed is:

a. 20 **b. 50**

c. 80 d. None of the above

39. Width of a double row tail to tail barn is:

a. 8.5 m **b. 11.5 m**

c. 15.5 m d. None of the above

40. A dairy cows daily needs drinking water of about:

a. 30- 35 litre **b. 60- 80 litre**

c. 100-110 litre d. None of the above

41. The maximum THI in the dairy barn/shed should be:

a. 45 **b. 70**

c. 100 d. None of the above

42. Solid dung should be removed from the shed:

a. Once a week **b. Twice a day**

c. Alternate day d. None of the above

43. Disinfectant action of sunlight is due to:

a. Infrared rays **b. Ultra violet rays**

c. X-rays d. None of the above

44. Covered floor space requirement for a cow in LH system is:

a. 2.5 Sq.mt. **b. 3.5 Sq.mt.**

c. 7.5 Sq.mt. d. None of the above

45. Maximum number of calves kept in a calf pen is:

a. 10 **b. 20**

c. 40 d. None of the above

46. The zoological name of poultry is:

a. Chicken indiana b. Gallus indiana

c. Gallus domesticus d. Gallus europeans

47. Central Sheep and Wool Research Institute (CSWRI) is located at:

a. Avikanagar (Rajasthan) b. Makhdoom (UP)

c. Jodhpur (Rajasthan) d. Jaipur (Rajasthan)

48. National Research Centre (NRC) on camel is located at:

a. Jaipur b. Ahmedabad

c. Surat **d. Bikaner**

49. Animal behaviour is governed by:

a. Genes only b. Environment only

c. Genes and environment bothd. None of the above

50. Sick animals express following symptoms:

a. Dull eyes

b. Decrease in feed and fodder intake

c. Decrease in production

d. All of the above

51. Four teeth state (2 pairs) in goats refers to which age:
    a. 1 year **b. 2 years**
    c. 3 years d. 4 years

52. "Ivermectin" is a choice of drug for:
    a. Internal parasites b. External parasites
    c. Both of the above d. None of the above

53. Required brooding temperature in brooder houses for day old chicks is:
    a. 90^0 F b. 85^0 F
    c. 80^0 F d. 75^0 F

54. The optimum level of litter material (in inches) for deep litter system is:
    a. 1 b. 2
    c. 3 **d. 4**

55. Early sexual maturity of chicks can be achieved if the chicks are provided with:
    a. Shorter photo periods **b. Longer photo periods**
    c. No effect of photo period d. Less than 6 hrs photo period

56. Housing aspect in pet animal care has:
    a. Very little importance **b. Very high importance**
    c. No importance d. None of the above

57. Construction material for pig houses should be:
    a. Cheap and fireproof b. Easily available
    c. Non allergic to animals **d. None of the above**

58. Drinking water should be available in animal houses during:
    a. Day time b. Night
    c. Whole day d. Not required at all

59. Vermin-composting is based on:
    a. Animal farm waste b. Cow urine
    c. Non palatable meat bi-products d. None of the above

60. Biogas is made from:

    a. Dung | b. Cow urine
    c. Non palatable meat byproduct | d. None of the above

61. The largest breed of goat in India is:

    a. Beetal | b. Black Bengal
    c. Jamnapari | d. Kashmiri

62. The term dual purpose describes cattle that are:

    a. Two colors | **b. For milk and draught**
    c. For high milk yield and fat | d. None of the above

63. One cubic meter can store manure:

    a. 5.0 Qtls. | **b. 4.5 Qtls.**
    c. 4.0 Qtls. | d. 3.5 Qtls.

64. Pitch angle of roof should not exceed:

    a. 30^0 | b. 40^0
    c. $\mathbf{45^0}$ | d. 35^0

65. The evaporative heat loss in buffaloes is:

    a. Poor | b. Good
    c. Medium | d. None of the above

66. Floor space requirement per bird of 0-8 weeks of age is:

    a. 900 cm^2 | **b. 700** $\mathbf{cm^2}$
    c. 800 cm^2 | d. 850 cm^2

67. In India green fodder availabiliy is:

    a. 673 million tones | **b. 573.5 million tones**
    c. 493.4 million tones | d. None of the above

68. Concentrate contains crude fibre:

    a. Less than 20 percent | **b. More than 18** percent
    c. Less than 18 percent | d. More than 20 percent

69. Wilting should be done to maintain dry matter:

a. 30-35 percent | b. 35-40 percent
c. 25-30 percent | d. 20-25 percent

70. Top of silo pit should be covered with wheat straw/rice straw layer of thickness:

a. 5-10 cm | b. 10-15 cm
c. 15-20 cm | d. 12-15 cm

71. Sweet dark brown silage is produced when temperature rises to:

a. 30-40^{0}C | **b. 35-40^{0}C**
c. 40-45^{0}C | d. 45-50^{0}C

72. Seed rate of bajra per hectare is:

a. 2-5 – 6 kg | b. 7.5 – 10 kg
c. 5.0 – 7.5 kg | d. 6.5 – 9.0 kg

73. Teat dipping is done for:

a. Proper let down | b. More milk
c. Preventing mastitis | d. None of the above

74. Foaling is the act of giving birth in:

a. Sow | **b. Mare**
c. Camel | d. None of the above

75. The carcass must be deeply buried with lime powder in which of the following disease:

a. FMD | **b. Anthrax**
c. Milk fever | d. None of the above

76. The ideal dairy cow must have following number of wedges:

a. 4 wedges | b. 2 wedges
c. 1 wedge | d. None of the above

77. The best method of milking a cow is:

a. Fisting | b. Knuckling
c. Stripping | d. None of the above

78. The buffalo having copper coloured skin and high fat content in milk is:

a. Murrah **b. Bhadawari**

c. Nilliravi d. None of the above

79. Leguminous fodders are rich source of:

a. Energy **b. Protein**

c. Fibre d. None of the above

80. The per acre seed rate of barseem is:

a. 4 kg **b. 10 kg**

c. 20 kg d. None of the above

81. The appropriate stage of harvesting maize fodder crop is:

a. Dough stage b. Milk stage

c. Mature stage d. None of the above

82. Stocking density is how many times more than the carrying capacity of grazing lands in India:

a. 10 times **b. 30 times**

c. 50 times d. None of the above

83. The best fodder for silage making is:

a. Bajra b. Barseem

c. Maize fodder d. None of the above

84. The perennial fodder crop is:

a. Sorghum b. Oats

c. Hybrid Napier d. None of the above

85. The angle of roof pitch in heavy rainfall areas should be:

a. 45^0 b. 60^0

c. 30^0 d. None of the above

86. The maximum number of cows per shed in LH system is:

a. 30 **b. 50**

c. 75 d. None of the abov

87. The solution of chlorine used for rinsing teat cups is:

    a. 200 ppm b. 100 ppm
    c. 50 ppm d. None of the above

88. The quality of deep well water for animals is:

    a. Wholesome b. Suspicious
    c. Dangerous d. None of the above

90. Temporary hardness of water is due to:

    a. Bi-carbonates b. Calcium sulphate
    c. Magnesium chloride d. None of the above

91. The device used to check back flow of water in a drainage system is:

    a. Trap b. Band
    c. Joint d. None of the above

92. The hormone responsible for let down of milk of:

    a. Epinephrine **b. Oxytocin**
    c. Progesterone d. None of the above

93. The best method of identification of pigs:

    a. Tagging **b. Ear-notching**
    c. Hot-branding d. None of the above

94. Newly born calves should be fed colostrums of body weight:

    a. $1/5^{th}$ **b.** $\mathbf{1/10^{th}}$
    c. $1/15^{th}$ d. None of the above

95. Milking of cow should be completed within:

    a. 4- 5 min **b. 7- 8 min**
    c. 12-15 min d. None of the above

96. The body condition score of dairy heifers should be between :

    a. 1.0–1.5 **b. 2.5–3.0**
    c. 4.5–5.0 d. None of the above

97. The bullock of which breed is famous for sawai-chal :

a.	**Kankrej**	b	Hariana
c.	Nagore	d.	None of the above

98. Tick the temperature of electric dehorner used for disbudding :

a.	140^{0}C	b.	340^{0}C
c.	**540^{0}C**	d.	None of the above

99. Central pair of permanent incisors in cattle erupts at :

a.	5 years	b.	4 years
c.	**2 years**	d.	None of the above

100. The maximum depth of silo-pit should be :

a.	6 feet	**b.**	**10 feet**
c.	20 feet	d.	None of the above

101. One acre of fodder land is sufficient for how many cross bred cows:

a.	2	**b.**	**4**
c.	8	d.	None of the above

102. Inoculation of fodder seed required for:

a.	Oats	**b.**	**Barseem**
c.	Sorghum	d.	None of the above

103. The hybrid Napier gives fodder throughout the year except at:

a.	Summer	**b.**	**Winter**
c.	Rainy season	d.	None of the above

104. The best summer legume fodder is:

a.	MP Chari	b.	Barseem
c.	**Cow pea**	d.	None of the above

105. Central zone in exotic cattle is:

a.	10-32^{0}C	**b.**	**13-18^{0}C**
c.	25-37^{0}C	d.	None of the above

106. The orientation of dairy shed in tropics should be in:

a. **East-West** b. North-South

c. North-West d. None of the above

107. The acceptable threshold limit for ammonia in dairy barn is:

a. 10 ppm **b.** **50 ppm**

c. 75 ppm d. None of the above

108. The angle of tilted roof pitch should be:

a. **30^0** b. 45^0

c. 75^0 d. None of the above

109. The open area for buffalos in LH system provided is:

a. **8 square meter** b. 10 square meter

c. 20 square meter d. None of the above

110. Number of dairy heifers per shed should be:

a. **20** b. 30

c. 50 d. None of the above

111. A newly born buffalo calf has got:

a. Four stomach **b.** **Simple stomach**

c. Developed rumen d. None of the above

112. Normally a cow calf immediately after its birth starts searching the teat of its dam within:

a. 5.0 hrs. b. 1.0 hrs

c. **2.0 hrs** d. None of the above

113. The ideal dry period in cow is:

a. 100 days b. 200days

c. **60 days** d. 30 days

114. Timely colostrum feeding is helpful for calves in:

a. Standing **b.** **Disease protection**

c. Rumination d. Sleeping

115. The distinct character of Nilliravi buffalo is:

a. Its sickle shape horn b. Blue colour

c. Five white patch on body d. Long hairs

116. The optimum temperature of milk for feeding cow calves is:

a. 36-39^{0}C b. 10-13^{0}C

c. 20-23^{0}C d. None of the above

117. The angle between earth and the ramp for loading pigs should be:

a. 85^0 - 90^0 b. 45^0 - 50^0

c. 15^0 – 20^0 d. None of the above

118. Pregnant animals should be fed adequately to gain significant body weight in last phase of gestation and it is called as:

a. Heating up b. Warming up

c. Steaming up d. None of the above

122. Air volume required per cow per hour is:

a. 400 cubit feet **b. 4000 cubic feet**

c. 36 cubic feet d. None of the above

123. The water is called hard due to :

a. Calcium salts b. Copper salts

c. Selenium d. None of the above

124. The quantity of dung voided by one adult cattle daily is:

a. 25-27 kg **b. 15-16 kg**

c. 5-6 kg d. None of the above

125. Hollow blocks are made of :

a. Bricks b. Plastic

c. Cement, concrete and sand d. None of the above

126. Akra walling is prevalent in hills for:

a. Cattle houses **b. Poultry houses**

c. Pig house d. None of the above

127. The depth of cattle feeding trough in loose housing system should be:

a. 80 cm | **b. 40 cm**

c. 20 cm | d. None of the above

128. The proportion of feeding trough and water trough in loose housing system should be:

a. 1:10 | b. 1:20

c. 1:25 | d. None of the above

129. Slope of concrete standing floor should be:

a. 1: 100 | b. 1: 60

c. 1: 40 | d. None of the above

130. The mixture of legume and non-legume green fodder is necessary for :

a. Providing enough crude fibre

b. Providing nutrients in proper ratio

c. Increasing energy value

d. None of the above

131. The ideal height of grasses in pasture for grazing of buffaloes:

a. 15 cm | b. 50 cm

c. 10 cm | d. None of the above

132. The average seed rate of oats (kg/hectare) is:

a. 30 kg | b. 15 kg

c. **80 kg** | d. None of the above

133. The S.S.G. is grown by:

a. Seed | b. Root cutting

c. Stem cutting | d. None of the above

134. The ideal time for lucerne sowing in Indian plain is:

a. July–August | b. March

c. December-January | **d. None of the above**

135. In barseem sowing the following should be added as mix crop:

a. Sorghum
b. Hybrid bajra
c. Chinese cabbage
d. None of the above

136. Hybrid Napier should be planted during :

a. June – July
b. October – November
c. December – January
d. None of the above

137. Sheep attain their full growth at the average age of:

a. 1 year
b. 2 years
c. 3 years
d. 4 years

138. The optimum age for breeding ram is from:

a. 1 to 2½ years
b. $2^{1/2}$ to 7 years
c. 7 to 9 years
d. 9 to 12 years

139. Gestation period in sheep is:

a. 87 days
b. 117 days
c. 147 days
d. 177 days

140. One ram can be used in a year for natural mating of:

a. 3 to 4 eves
b. 30 to 40 eves
c. 300 to 400 eves
d. 600 to 800 eves

141. Sheep love to stay:

a. In highly crowded sheds
b. In medium crowded sheds
c. In uncrowned sheds
d. Under open skies

142. Exotic breed of goat is:

a. Saanen
b. Beetal
c. Osmanabadi
d. Surti

143. In goat heat occurs at an interval of:

a. 7 to 8 days
b. 17 to 18 days
c. 27 to 28 days
d. 37 to 38 days

144. Fresh air contains carbon dioxide to the extent of approximately:

a. 0.028 - 0.04 percent
b. 0.28 - 0.4 percent
c. 2.8 - 4.00 percent
d. 28 - 40 percent

145. Pure air contains nitrogen to the extent of approximately:

a. 18.04 percent
b. 38.04 percent
c. 58.04 percent
d. 78.04 per cent

146. Which one of the following animals excretes maximum CO_2 hourly:

a. Horses
b. Swine
c. Cows in milk
d. Sheep

147. The building for housing animals in a large agricultural farm should be constructed near the:

a. Northern corner of the farm
b. Centre of the farm
c. Eastern corner of the farm
d. Southern or western corner of the farm

148. The animal building may be constructed in the shape of the letters L, U, T or E with a road round the outside, the open end of the letters facing:

a. North
b. South
c. East
d. West

149. For plastering inner or outer surface of walls, cement plaster consisting of clean, sharp sand and portland cement respectively is used by mixing in which one of the following proportions:

a. 8:1
b. 6:1
c. 4:1
d. 2:1

150. Except at a very great cost, it is impossible to get perfect timber for building purposes of the defects in timber, which one of the following when present in undue proportion is the most serious:

a. Shakes
b. Knotes
c. Dry rot
d. Sapwood

151. Which one of the following is the softest water:

a. Rain water
b. River water
c. Spring water
d. Deep well water

152. Hydraulic test is done for:

a. Testing of drains
b. Softening of water
c. Purification of sewage
d. None of the above

153. On the basis of agricultural and animal husbandry regions of India, the map of the agricultural and animal husbandry zones of India is divided into:

a. 5 zones
b. 10 zones
c. 15 zones
d. 20 zones

154. The rain fall in Tarai areas of Uttar Pradesh/Uttarakhand is about:

a. 4 inches
b. 20 inches
c. 40 inches
d. 80 inches

155. The major grassland type found in Tarai areas of U.P. is:

a. Brothriochloa
b. Phragmites/Saharum
c. Cymbopogon
d. Arundinella

156. In a drainage system the slope should be one in every:

a. 60 inches
b. 40 inches
c. 80 inches
d. 30 inches

157. Dairy cow should be provided air space of cubic feet:

a. 200
b. 600
c. 400
d. 800

158. Indian cattle maintain their body temperature through:

a. Abdomen
b. Dewlap
c. Tail
d. Hair

159. Gestation period in water buffalo is:

a. 10 months and 10 days
b. 12 months and 12 days
c. 11 months and 11 days
d. 9 months and 9 days

160. Pashmina is obtained from:

a.	**Goat**	b.	Sheep
c.	Rabbit	d.	Yak

161. Approximate weight newborn cow's calf is:

a.	27-18 kg	b.	15-20 kg
c.	**20-25 kg**	d.	30-32 kg

162. Urea contains what percent of nitrogen:

a.	40 %	**b.**	**46 %**
c.	36 %	d.	56 %

163. Heat cycle comes in ewes after days:

a.	20-22	b.	23-25
c.	**17-19**	d.	15-16

164. Gestation period in mare is:

a.	280 - 290 days	b.	150 - 160 days
c.	**336 - 340 days**	d.	310 - 320 days

165. The seed rate of barseem per hectare is:

a.	50 kg	**b.**	**25 kg**
c.	45 kg	d.	60 kg

166. Silvi pasture consists of:

a.	Trees alone	b.	Grasses alone
c.	**Grasses and trees**	d.	None of the above

167. M.P.Chari is the variety of:

a.	Barseem	b.	Lucerne
c.	**Sorghum**	d.	Bajra

168. The anti-quality content of lucerne is:

a.	**Nitrate**	b.	HCV
c.	Saponin	d.	Mimosure

169. Optimum temperature for sowing of berseem is:

a.	**20-25°C**	b.	30-35°C
c.	15-20°C	d.	None of the above

170. Which of the following is water borne disease caused by a virus:

a.	Black quarter	b.	Anthrax
c.	**Foot and mouth disease**	d.	Amoebiasis

Q.3. Fill up the blanks:

1. Adult female of goat is called ***doe.***
2. Colour of the Jersey breed is ***red.***
3. Best method of identification in sheep is ***tagging.***
4. Newly born calves should be fed colostrum at least for ***3*** days.
5. Wallowing during ***summer*** season is beneficial for buffaloes.
6. ***Jaffarabadi*** is the heaviest breed of Indian buffalo.
7. Animal can lose all ***fat and 50% protein*** and may still remain alive.
8. Water makes about ***70 %*** of animals body weight.
9. In hot weather animal consumes more water because of ***heat stress***.
10. The height of manure pit should not be more than ***1.5 to 2.0 m***.
11. Sheep and goat void dung in the form of ***small globules.***
12. A cow inhales ***3.13 m^3*** air/hour.
13. Light prevents barns and houses from becoming ***mouldy.***
14. Growing animals require ***more*** water than adult animals.
15. Leguminous fodders are rich in ***protein.***
16. Scarcity of green fodder occurs in two periods during the year i.e. ***June*** and ***October.***
17. To obtain more nutrients per unit of land the crop should be harvested at ***preflowering*** for hay making.
18. In rotational deferred grazing system, the whole plot is divided into ***4 parts.***

19. The proportion of concentrate increases forage consumption is reduced to ***0.25 to 0.8 kg*** for each additional kg of concentrate consumed.
20. Legumes are very susceptible to ***salinity*** and ***alkalinity***
21. A cow apparently always in heat is called ***buller***.
22. Tallest breed of sheep in India is ***Nellore.***
23. The smallest piglet in a litter is called ***runt/crit***.
24. First faeces voided by a calf is called ***muconium.***
25. Freckles on the body and loopy ears are the breed character of ***Berkshire*** pigs.
26. Falling of animals, on the ground is called ***casting.***
27. The best method of identification in cattle is ***hot branding***.
28. The scientific name of anjan grass is ***Cenchrus ciliaris***.
29. Best time for harvesting maize fodder is ***milk stage.***
30. Nali sheep is famous for ***carpet wool*** production.
31. Best stage for harvesting of sorghum is ***dough*** stage.
32. Important legume fodder for summer and Kharif season is ***cowpea.***
33. The important perennial fodder crop is ***napier.***
34. The stocking density in Indian pastures is commonly more than ***10*** times.
35. Four crossbred cows can be maintained on one acre of fodder land.
36. The pitch angle of asbestos sheet of roof should be ***15-18^0.***
37. Adult cattle requires about ***3500-4000*** cubic ft. fresh air per hour.
38. Disease control is ***difficult*** in loose housing system.
39. Opening which allows the escape of foul air is known as ***outlet/exhaust.***
40. The desirable slope in barn floors should be ***1 inch*** for every 60 inches.
41. The pitch angle of tiled roof should be ***25-30^{0}C.***
42. Hay from oats is prepared during ***summer*** season.
43. Lush green fodder is essential for ***dairy*** animals.
44. Most of the fodder grasses are ***perennial*** in nature.
45. ***Dung*** is the main animal waste of dairy farms.

46. Meadows are natural ***grass land*** situated in temperate regions.
47. ***Tree lopping*** is the main fodder resource in arid regions.
48. Cowpea is fed to animals during ***summer*** season
49. Surplus fodder may be preserved for ***lean*** periods, if any.
50. Large dairy farms of India generally prefer ***loose*** type of animal housing system.
51. Cost of animal house increases with ***increase*** in the size of operating unit.
52. India could be divided into ***5*** agro-climatic zones from the viewpoint of animal production.
53. Tail to tail system is ***better*** than head to head system of housing.
54. ***Fast*** growing dense trees should be planted in/around animal farm.
55. Floor of animal houses should be non ***slippery*** in nature.
56. ***Temperature / rainfall / humidity / solar radiation*** are the essential components of climate of an area.
57. Proper ***ventilation*** is required for avoiding diseases and to optimize production.
58. Number of incisor teeth in the lower jaw of an adult ox are ***eight.***
59. Buffalo belongs to the family ***bovidae.***
60. Single humped camel is called ***dromedary.***
61. Large litter size is found in ***swine.***
62. Dairy cow should have ***wedge*** shape body.
63. Act of mating in sheep is known as ***tupping.***
64. Best crop for silage making in ***Kharif*** season is maize.
65. At present only ***6-7 million*** hectares of land falls under fodder crops.
66. Crops which last for many years are called ***permanent pasture.***
67. Native pastures are those which grow in area where average rain fall is ***20 inches.***
68. Feed constitute is about ***70 %*** of the maintenance cost.
69. Average yield of hybrid napier is ***600 Qtls*** per hectare.

70. The pigs of ***Large White Yorkshire*** breed have erect ears and curling tail.
71. Gestation period in case of pigs is ***112-114*** days.
72. Mule is a hybrid between ***Jack*** and ***Mare.***
73. Colostrum should be provided to newly born calf within ***2 hours*** of birth.
74. One skilled milker is allotted ***12*** milch cows in hand milking system.
75. The meat of pig is called ***pork.***
76. The best age of disbudding a calf is ***7-12*** days of age.
77. The incubation period for chiken egg is ***21*** days.
78. The barseem seed should be inoculated with ***rhizobium*** before sowing.
79. One assumed cattle unit is equal to ***5*** sheep/goat.
80. The maximum depth of a silo pit should be ***10 feet.***
81. On one acre good fodder land ***4*** cross bred cows can be raised.
82. ***11000*** of root cuttings are required for planting hybrid napier in one acre.
83. The per acre seed rate of oat fodder is ***35-40*** kg.
84. ***Lucerne*** is a good legume perennial fodder crop.
85. The orientation of dairy buildings should be in ***east & west*** direction.
86. The covered area and open area provided to dairy cows is ***3.5*** and ***7.0*** square metre in LH system.
87. Dairy cow needs air space of about ***22.5*** cubic meters.
88. The acceptable threshold limit for ammonia in a dairy barn is ***50*** ppm.
89. The angle of roof pitch should be ***25.30^{0}*** in tiled roof shed.
90. There should be ***1*** inch slope for every ***40*** inch of length from front to back in floors.
91. The TNZ range in zebu cattle is ***10-32^{0}C.***
92. Special poultry birds raise for meat purpose are called ***broilers.***
93. Gestation period in case of buffalo is ***310*** days.
94. ***Nali*** is the best breed of sheep famous for carpet wool production.
95. ***Ear notching*** is the best method of identification in pigs.

96. A vasectomized bull is called ***teaser***.

97. The scientific name of buffalo is ***Bubalus bubalis***

98. The first milk immediately after calving is called ***colostrum.***

99. The goat breed which is prolific, gives birth to 3-4 kids in a litter is ***Black Bengal***.

100. Indian pastures are seriously lacking ***perennial legume*** grasses.

101. The harvesting stage of maize fodder is ***milk*** *stage*.

102. On one acre good fodder land ***5*** buffalo as can be raised.

103. Lucerne gives fodder throughout the year except ***rainy season***.

104. Seed rate of barseem is ***10-12*** kg per acre.

105. The numbers of root cuttings/stem cuttings required for planting hybrid Napier are ***11000*** cutting.

106. The stage of harvesting cow pea fodder is ***seed pod stage.***

107. ***Over/continuous*** grazing is the major problem of Indian grazing lands.

108. Methane level is toxic @ ***50000*** ppm in shed.

109. The water requirement per cow is ***60-80*** litres/day.

110. The acceptable limit of CO_2 is ***5000*** ppm in cow shed.

111. One square feet of window space is given for ***30*** square feet of floor area.

112. Hardness in water due to ***Calcium sulphate*** is called permanent hardness.

113. The most common method of testing drain pipes is ***smoke/water***.

114. There is more problem of bossy cows in ***LH system*** housing system.

115. One person can milk ***12-14*** cows both times daily.

116. A common liver parasite usually found in marshy places is ***liver fluke***.

117. The balance used for recording milk of cows is called as ***herd recorder***.

118. The pendulous body between the fore limbs of buffaloes is called as ***brisket***.

119. The fluid flowing in milk vein is ***blood***.

120. Parturition in swine is called as ***farrowing***.

121. The depth of dipping tank for pigs should be ***100*** cm.

122. The chemical used for chemical dehorning is ***sodium hydroxide/***

potassium hydroxide

123. ***Poultry*** manure is the richest of all.
124. A neutral or slightly alkaline pH between ***7-7.5*** is considered to be best for compositing.
125. Approximately ***100 to 150*** g excreta is available per bird per day with 25% solid in it.
126. Poultry manure having more than ***30%*** moisture content can not be stored without further aeration if mal-odours are to be prevented.
127. The flow of water in a drain depends upon the ***slope*** of the drain.
128. A satisfactory trap must effectively ***prevent*** sewer gases into inlet pipes.
129. One adult cow requires about ***60*** litres of drinking water daily in the summer.
130. The scientific name of the house fly is ***Musca domestica.***
131. P.C. 6 is a variety of ***sorghum.***
132. Mescavy is a variety of ***barseem.***
133. Hara sona is a variety of ***SSG (multi-cut jawar).***
134. Maize + ***lobia (cow-pea)*** can be cultivated almost around the year in Indian plains.
135. Forage tree leaves have got high content of ***tannin/lignin*** which is an anti-nutritional actor.
136. The pH of good silage is ***4.0.***
137. The ideal moisture content of hay is ***10-12 percent.***
138. The hybrid Napier can be inter-cropped with ***barseem or lucerne*** during winter.
139. The highest sheep population is found in the state of ***Rajasthan.***
140. The face of Chokla breed of sheep of Rajasthan is of ***dark brown*** colour
141. ***Nellore*** is the tallest breed of sheep in india resembling goat in appearence.
142. The smallest breed of goat in India is ***Black Bengal.***
143. ***Muzzafarnagari*** is the sheep breed of West U.P.
144. Face of Russian Merino is of ***white*** colour.
145. Normal life span of sheep is ***12-14*** years.

146. Term humidity refers to the amount of ***water*** vapor present in atmosphere.
147. The expired air of herbivorous animals, in addition to O_2, CO_2 and N_2 also contains considerable amount of ***methane*** derived from carbohydrate fermentation in the alimentary canal.
148. Damp floors and ***damp*** walls are marked predisposing causes of illness and general debility.
149. Ordinary building bricks are comparatively soft and wear very unevenly if used for ***flooring.***
150. Pipes for underground drains must possess ***strength*** to withstand the pressure of the superimposed soil and the weight of traffic.
151. The housing required for calves depends on whether they are to be hand fed or ***weaned.***
152. ***Hard*** water has been held responsible for development of goiter and renal calculi.
153. In spite of scientific proof to the contrary, many dairymen persistently hold the erroneous opinion that warmth is necessary for ***more*** production.
154. Gestation period of sow is ***114*** days.
155. Pica is due to deficiency of ***phosphorus.***
156. Excellent milk producing breed of buffalo is ***Murrah.***
157. Best method of identification in pigs is ***ear notching***.
158. Best draught breed of camel is ***Bikaneri***.
159. Act of parturition in mare is ***foaling.***
160. Central Avian Research Institute (CARI) is situated at ***Izatnagar.***
161. In which buffalo breed, coat colour is copper like ***Bhadawari.***
162. Feed having high DCP and TDN percent is known as ***concentrate***.
163. Bloat is caused by excessive feeding of ***green fodder***.
164. The anti-quality content of sorghum is ***HCN.***
165. The pH of good silage is ***3.5 to 4.2***.
166. Which fodder crop is suitable for hay making ***lucerne.***
167. Crops should contain an adequate level of sugar and starch for ***acid fermentation.***

168. The seed rate of barley per hectare is ***100*** kg.

169. One gram of dry matter yields ***4.4 k cal*** of energy.

170. Prolonged inhalation of carbon mono oxide at low concentration causes ***anemia.***

171. There must be a ***gully trap*** between drain and sewer.

172. The space requirement for broiler is ***one square feet.***

173. Under loose housing system, covered area required per buffalo is ***4 square metre.***

174. ***Nitrosomonas*** bacteria convert ammonia radicals into nitrites.

175. One milli equivalent per litre of hardness producing ion is equal to ***50 ppm*** of $CaCO_3$.

9

Livestock Producton & Management (PART-II) Production and Management of Swine, Sheep, Goat, Equine & Camel

Q.1. True or False:

1. True — The foal attains double its weight one month after birth.
2. True — In camel there is clear cut demarcation line between vulva and vagina.
3. False — The sow moves during standing heat when the back is pressed.
4. False — Group of horse is termed as herd.
5. False — The animal should be excited before slaughter.
6. True — Flushing increases the number of ova.
7. False — National research centre on equine is located at Bikaner.
8. False — Creep ration should have 14-15% protein.
9. False — Dipping should be done in rainy season.
10. True — Prolificacy of Black Bengal is very high.
11. True — Karakul is a pelt producing breed.
12. True — Methionine is a sulphur containing amino acid.
13. False — Beetal breed of goat belongs to Baitul district of M.P.
14. True — Docking in sheep reduces the parasitic infestation.
15. False — Nibbling is a habit of goat.

16.	True	Sheep belongs to family bovidae.
17.	True	The height of A-class horse is 15 hands or more.
18.	False	Freckles are more common in Berkshire pigs.
19.	True	Exercise bandages are applied on cannon between knee and fetlock.
20.	True	The gallop is a 4 beat gait.
21.	True	A bay horse usually has black points on mane, tail, limbs and tip of ears.
22.	True	A flute bit is commonly applied in horses to prevent wind sucking vice.
23.	False	Never provide moderate exercise to mare just after foaling.
24.	True	The cow camel has follicular cycle in the estrus period.
25.	True	Shortness and fineness of wool fibre are associated.
26.	False	Wool is the least hygroscopic fibre.
27.	True	Pure fine wool has non-medulated fibres.
28.	False	The suint is insoluble in water.
29.	True	Goats of alpine breed have perky ears.
30.	False	If difference between staple length and fibre length is more, the wool is coarse.
31.	True	The feed and water intake increases after shearing.
32.	True	Copper deficiency is associated with steely wool production.
33.	True	The camel breeds only in winter months i.e. during November to March.
34.	False	A pig may be fed minimum of concentrate and maximum of roughages.
35.	False	The feed, labour and housing cost for a sow with 2 pigs will be different from a sow with 10 pigs.
36.	True	Mature male horse has total 40 teeth whereas young horse has 24 teeth.
37.	True	The hump in camel is nothing but a lump of fat which serves as a reservoir of energy during lean period.

38.	True	Cross bred pigs can increase litter size, livability but not carcass traits.
39.	True	Horses sleep while standing.
40.	True	A pregnant she camel cocks her tail at the approach of man or a male camel is the best and easiest method to detect pregnancy.
41.	True	Goat is the most prolific of all domesticated ruminants under tropical and subtropical conditions.
42.	True	Chain linked fencing is the best for sheep and goat.
43.	False	The feeding of sheep in stall is more economic than grazing on pasture.
44.	True	Breeding male kids should always be kept separate from 4 month onwards.
45.	False	Sheep and goat are monogastric animals.
46.	False	All young male kids meant for breeding should be castrated at two and half months of age.
47.	False	The convenient time for dipping is shortly before shearing.
48.	True	Most widely practiced system of mating is to run rams with ewes during mating seasons.
49.	False	The habitat of Polland China breed of swine is Beijing.
50.	True	The ratio of male and female in a camel herd is 1:15-30.
51.	False	Hybrid whose sire is stallion and dam is jannet is known as mule.
52.	False	Swine fever is a bacterial disease.
53.	True	The age of weaning in foal is six months.
54.	False	Anvil is a instrument used in grooming.
55.	True	National research centre of camel is situated at Bikaner.
56.	True	Ruting in camel is denoted as breeding season.
57.	True	Pashmina has more insulating value than fine wool.
58.	True	Karakul breed of sheep is famous for pelt production.
59.	False	More is the medulla percentage, finer is the wool.
60.	True	Black Bengal is a highly prolific breed of goat.

61.	True	Mandya is the best mutton purpose breed of sheep in India.
62.	False	Lanameter is used for recording of grazing time.
63.	True	The water requirement of goat is double the dry matter requirement.
64.	False	Mandya is the largest breed of goat.
65.	True	There are 6 incisor teeth in a horse.
66.	False	The gestation period of mule is 336 days.
67.	False	Winking is a symptom of heat in swine.
68.	False	Landrace is a native of U.K.
69.	True	Flushing is generally done two weeks before breeding.
70.	False	In mares, postpartum oestrous is also called as dioestrous.
71.	True	Camel possesses 34 numbers of permanent teeth.
72.	False	*Camelus dromedarius* is the zoological name of double humped camel.
73.	True	Six to ten months year old sheep possess four pairs of incisors.
74.	True	At 28 months of age, in sheep the 3rd pair of incisor becomes permanent.
75.	False	The normal birth weight of lamb varies from 1.5 to 2 kg.
76.	False	Hand shear is an instrument used for grooming.
77.	True	Ballotment of belly from three months onward is a method to diagnose pregnancy in goat.
78.	True	At 6 months age 25 kg body weight of kid is good for slaughter purposes.
79.	True	An average goat (in milk) requires 3.5 to 4.5 kg fodder per day.
80.	False	In yak, the thoracic ribs are present in 13 pairs.
81.	False	Regurgitation is not common in camel.
82.	True	The tail of healthy pigs is usually curled.
83.	True	The fat from a boar is known as lard.
84.	True	Space requirement for a breeding boar is 1 metre wide by 1.5 metre long.

85. False The front arch of the saddle is known as pommel.

86. True Ear notching is a common method of identification in pigs.

87. True The housing of swine is called sty.

88. True Plucking of undercoat is termed as rooing.

89. False Medullation percentage in Merino wool is maximum.

90. True Barbari and Black Bengal goats have kidding throughout the year.

91. True Selection of sheep for wool production may be done at the age of weaning to reduce the cost of rearing.

92. True Jamnapari is the tallest and heaviest breed of Indian goats.

93. False Ram marking is a method of identification of adult male sheep.

94. True Synchronization of estrus in sheep is performed by hormonal intravaginal insert device.

95. False Pigs are weaned at one week of age.

96. True Pigs above 60 kg live weight are known as finishing pigs.

97. True Camel can tolerate a loss of water at about 30 per cent of its body weight.

98. False In equine, RBC retains excess body water for emergency.

99. False Bacterian camel is a single humped camel.

100. True The average gestation period of mare is 340 days.

101. False Flushing is generally practiced in mares.

102. False Seggy is a ram castrated before service.

103. True A worthless lamb is called skip.

104. False Hissardale is a mutton breed of sheep.

105. True Kashmiri is one of the fibre type breed of goat.

106. True Ganjam is a breed of south Orissa.

107. False Saanen is also known as Jersey cow of the world.

108. True Muzaffarnagri is a sheep breed of U.P.

109. True Rambouillet was developed in France.

Q.2. Multiple Choices :

1. The size of corpora lutea in swine is:

   a. 1 inch b. 1½ inch

   c. 2 inch d. 5 inch

2. The average calving interval of camel ranges from:

   a. 500-600 days **b. 700-800 days**

   c. 365-400 days d. None of the above

3. The height of pony should be less than:

   a. 13 feet **b. 14 hand**

   c. 13 meter d. None of the above

4. Number of chromosome in camel is:

   a. 74 b. 60

   c. 62 d. 56

5. While selecting gilt the back fat thickness should be less than:

   a. 4 cm b. 10 cm

   c. 6 cm d. None of the above

6. The dry matter requirement of adult camel is:

   a. 2 % of body weight b. 3.5 % of body weight

   c. 4 % of body weight d. 4 % of body weight

7. The camel does not have:

   a. Seminal vesicle b. Cowper's gland

   c. Prostate gland d. None of the above

8. The covered floor space requirement for lactating sow is:

   a. 70-80 sq. ft. b. 20-30 sq. ft.

   c. 40-50 sq. ft. d. None of the above

9. Milk of goat is very digestible because:

   a. Small size of fat globule b. More fat contents

   c. More protein contents d. None of the above

10. Neonatal ataxia in lamb is due to the deficiency of:

a.	Ca	b.	P
c.	**Cu**	d.	Na

11. Diameter of fine wool should be less than:

a.	**18 micron**	b.	30 micron
c.	25 micron	d.	None of the above

12. Crossbred of Malpura and Dorset is known as:

a.	**Mutton synthetic**	b.	Bharat Merino
c.	Avivastra	d.	Hissardale

13. Kathiawari sheep belongs to:

a.	Rajasthan	**b.**	**Gujarat**
c.	Madhya Pradesh	d.	Himachal Pradesh

14. Fine wool producing breed of sheep is:

a.	**Rambouillet**	b.	Bikaneri
c.	Kutchi	d.	Pattanwari

15. Common colour of Barbari goat is:

a.	White	b.	Brown
c.	**White with brown patch**	d.	None of the above

16. Nilgiri breed of sheep was evolved from indigenous breed of :

a.	**Coimbatore**	b.	Gurej
c.	Jalauni	d.	None of the above

17. The canter is a characteristic gait having:

a.	2 beat gait	**b.**	**3-beat gait**
c.	4 beat gait	d.	None of the above

18. An isolated white mark between the nostrils in horse is called:

a.	Blaze	**b.**	**Snip**
c.	Spot	d.	Nonc of thc abovc

19. Tethering of red ribbon around tail is a conventional sign of:

    a. Kicker b. Biting
    c. Jibbing d. None of the above

20. The Forsell's operation gives good result in:

    a. Wind sucking b. Rearing
    c. Balking d. None of the above

21. Showing the white of eye should always be noted while writing soundness certificate:

    a. Kicking **b. Biting**
    c. Wind sucking d. None of the above

22. Cocking of tail is a pretty good diagnosis of pregnancy in:

    a. Sow b. Mare
    c. Cow camel d. None of the above

23. The orientation of goat sheds should be in the direction:

    a. North-South **b. East-West**
    c. South-North d. None of the above

24. The famous breed of sheep for pelt production is:

    a. Angora **b. Karakul**
    c. Nali d. None of the above

25. Indian goat breed which is a regular breeder:

    a. Jamnapari b. Beetal
    c. Barbari d. None of the above

26. The CSWRI is located near:

    a. Hissar b. Bikaner
    c. Malpura d. None of the above

27. The best time of feeding colostrum to newly born lamb is:

    a. Within half to one hour of birth
    b. 10-12 hours of birth
    c. After discharge of placenta
    d. None of the above

28. Which is the maximum coarse wool among the following:

a. 34 s b. 46 s

c. 64 s d. 80 s

29. The famous sheep breed for carpet wool production is:

a. Nilgiri **b. Nali**

c. Nellore d. None of the above

30. Small sized goat breed famous for prolification, triplets, quadruplets but with poor nursing ability is:

a. Beetal **b. Black Bengal**

c. Malabar d. None of the above

31. Places of habitation in horse is:

a. Byre b. Sty

c. Stable d. Pen

32. Number of needle/black teeth in a new born pig is:

a. 12 b. 6

c. 4 **d. 8**

33. National Research Centre on Camel is located at:

a. Hisar b. Mathura

c. Udaipur **d. Bikaner**

34. Population of pigs in India is about:

a. 8 million b. 9 million

c. 11 million d. 14 million

35. In mares the duration of estrus is:

a. 18-19 hours b. 24-36 hours

c. 40-48 hours **d. 4-8 days**

36. The best method of identification in pigs is:

a. Tagging **b. Ear notching**

c. Tattooing d. Cold branding

37. Most of the pre-weaning mortality in pigs is due to:

a. Killing by dam
b. Crushing by dam
c. Piglet anemia
d. Chilling

38. Under intensive management the camel calf is allowed suckling and is weaned at:

a. 10 months
b. 12 months
c. 15 months
d. 20 months

39. In natural state goat prefers:

a. Nibbling
b. Grazing
c. Browsing
d. Stall feeding

40. One breeding ram is sufficient for mating of:

a. 30 to 40 ewes
b. 40 to 50 ewes
c. 60 to 70 ewes
d. 100 to 110 ewes

41. The greater weight of wool is shorn at:

a. 1st shearing
b. 2nd shearing
c. 3rd shearing
d. 4th shearing

42. Which of the following ingredient is used to make the ration bulky for starter kids:

a. Wheat
b. Oats
c. Rice bran
d. Soyabean meal

43. Angora goats are famous for their:

a. Meat
b. Milk
c. Mohair
d. None of the above

44. Gestation period of goat is:

a. 90 days
b. 120 days
c. 150 days
d. 180 days

45. Which of the following country is having the largest population of goat:

a. Iraq
b. India
c. Indonesia
d. Turkey

46. Floor space requirement per ram according to ISI standard is:
    a. 1.5 sqm. **b. 3.4 sqm.**
    c. 5.5 sqm. d. 2.5 sqm.

47. Five number nails in horse denote:
    a. Five inch length
    b. Five pounds weight of 1000 nails
    c. Five centimeter length
    d. None of the above

48. The teat of camel has following number of orifice:
    a. One **b. Two**
    c. Three d. Four

49. Nose peg is used in controlling of:
    a. Swine **b. Camel**
    c. Horse d. None of the above

50. Piglet anemia is caused due to deficiency of:
    a. Sodium b. Potassium
    c. Iron d. All of the above

51. The country having highest population of pig is:
    a. India **b. China**
    c. Poland d. Russia

52. Dhaman heat in mare occurs after foaling:
    a. 7-14 days b. 40-60 days
    c. 60-90 days d. None of the above

53. Method of castration in piglet is:
    a. Open method b. Burdizzo castrater
    c. Elastrator d. All of the above

54. Disbudding is done by:
    a. KOH b. NaOH
    c. Electric dehorner **d. All of the above**

55. The crispness in wool fiber is due to arrangement of:

a. Ortho b. Para

c. Both a and b d. None of the above

56. The highest population of goat is found in:

a. Pakistan **b. India**

c. Bangladesh d. Srilanka

57. Bharat Merino is developed at:

a. Avikanagar b. Makhdoom

c. Hisar d. Bikaner

58. The strength of wool fibre is measured by:

a. Lanameter b. Vibro recorder

c. Instron tester d. None of the above

59. Sangamneri breed of goat is found in:

a. Maharashtra b. Bihar

c. M.P. d. U.P.

60. Mohair is obtained from:

a. Angora b. Kaghani

c. Lehri d. Nachi

61. Goat milk has:

a. More fat present than buffalo **b. Smallest fat globule**

c. Similar odour of cow d. None of the above

62. Galvayne's marks appear at one of the following years of age in horse:

a. 9 years **b. 10 years**

c. 11 years d. None of the above

63. One male camel can cover about following female camels in one breeding season:

a. 20 - 50 b. 5 -10

c. 40 -70 d. None of the above

64. During rut season, the soft palate comes out in:

a.	Boar	b.	Mare
c.	**Male camel**	d.	None of the above

65. In horses, natural, rapid, two beat diagonal gait is called:

a.	Walk	**b.**	**Trot**
c.	Gallop	d.	None of the above

66. Gestation period of swine averages about:

a.	280 days	b.	340 days
c.	**114 days**	d.	None of the above

67. The floor space requirement of boar pen is:

a.	**40 to 50 sq.ft.**	b.	60 to 80 sq.ft.
c.	30 to 40 sq.ft.	d.	None of the above

68. Castrated female pig is called:

a.	Sow	b.	Gilt
c.	**Spayed**	d.	None of the above

69. How many kids per doe are preferred:

a.	1	**b.**	**2**
c.	3	d.	None of the above

70. In which month of the year most milk goats breed:

a.	January – February	**b.**	**May – June**
c.	September – October	d.	None of the above

71. The heat period of goat is:

a.	28 hrs.	**b.**	**38 hrs.**
c.	48 hrs.	d.	None of the above

72. The gestation period in goat is:

a.	135 days	**b.**	**145 days**
c.	165 days	d.	None of the above

73. Goat meat is known as:

a. Mutton | **b. Chevon**
c. Copon | d. None of the above

74. The famous small goat for meat is:

a. Assam hill | b. Angora
c. Black Bengal | d. None of the above

75. One ram is enough for:

a. 10 ewes | **b. 30 ewes**
c. 50 ewes | d. None of the above

76. At what time the sheep is put on pastures:

a. Just after lambing | b. Just before lambing
c. Just before shearing | d. None of the above

77. National research centre on equines is located at:

a. Bikaner | b. Indore
c. Mathura | **d. Hisar**

78. The carrying capacity of a horse wagon in broad gauge is:

a. 2 | b. 1
c. 8 | d. 16

79. The fastest gait with four feet in horse is known as:

a. Gallop | b. Pace
c. Canter | d. Trot

80. Which of the following breed has six white spots:

a. Berkshire | b. Hampshire
c. Back portion | d. Tail

81. Which portion of the body has maximum hair growth in yak:

a. Neck | b. Ventral part of the body
c. Back portion | d. Tail

82. In camel, sexual glands are present in both the sexes:

a. **Behind the head** b. At inguinal region

c. At the base of the tail d. Elbow joint

83. Lean pork is:

a. **Only meat but no fat**

b. Only meat but no skin

c. Only meat but no bones

d. Meat with fat and skin together

84. The lion eye area is measured:

a. **After slaughter**

b. Before slaughter of animal

c. While selection the animal for slaughter

d. During sale of pork

85. Goat milk is richer in:

a. Iron **b. Zinc**

c. Chlorine d. Manganese

86. A pair of goat can be kept in a pen of size measuring:

a. 6 X 3 feet b. 8 X 2 feet

c. 5 X 2.5 feet d. 5 X 4 feet

87. Barbari nannies attain the age of puberty:

a. 14 month b. 18 month

c. 10 month d. 16 month

88. The exotic breed of goat is:

a. Alpine b. Rambouillet

c. Landrace d. Barbari

89. The inter lambing period in sheep is normally found:

a. 15-20 months b. 14-18 months

c. 13-15 months **d. 8-12 months**

90. Maximum number of animals in one ram pen:

a. 1 b. 2

c. 3 d. Any number

91. Wool blindness is common in:

a. Merino b. Cheviot

c. Patanwari d. Marwari

92. Removal of burrs can be done by:

a. Cutting of fibers with scissors b. Beating the wool

c. Deburring machine **d. All of the above**

93. Average gestation period of camel is:

a. 280 days b. 340 days

c. 370 days d. None of the above

94. The finisher ration of pig contains:

a. 10 % protein b. 12 % protein

c. 13 % protein d. None of the above

95. In mares, the average duration of oestrus is:

a. 2 days b. 3 days

c. 5 days d. None of the above

96. Winking is a symptom of heat in :

a. Swine **b. Equine**

c. Camel d. None of the above

97. Landrace breed is a native of:

a. U.K. b. U.S.A.

c. France d. None of the above

98. Manipuri is an Indian breed of:

a. Pig **b. Horse**

c. Camel d. None of the above

99. The stallion requires an exercise of:

a. 30 min. daily | b. 1 hr. daily

c. 1 hr. 30 min. daily | d. None of the above

100. Grooming is generally practiced in:

a. Swine | **b. Equine**

c. Camel | d. None of the above

101. Lambs are castrated at:

a. 4 weeks of age | b. 3 weeks of age

c. 2 weeks of age | d. None of the above

102. Docking in dogs is preferred at:

a. 4 weeks of age | b. 3 weeks of age

c. 2 weeks of age | d. None of the above

103. A coarse and brittle wool fiber is called:

a. Fleece | **b. Kemp**

c. Wool | d. None of the above

104. Natural waviness of a fiber is called:

a. Kemp | **b. Crimp**

c. Lock | d. None of the above

105. The wool of pure merino has a spinning count of:

a. 64 s | b. 58 s

c. 44 s | d. None of the above

106. Secretion of sweat gland mostly of alkaline nature having potassium salt is:

a. Suint | b. Wax

c. Grease | d. None of the above

107. The home tract of Angora goat is:

a. Germany | **b. Turkey**

c. India | d. None of the above

108. Sheep are generally shorn:

  a. After the end of winter season

  b. At the beginning of winter season

  c. After the end of summer season

  d. None of the above

Q.3. Fill up the Blanks :

1. Needle teeth in pig are cut at ***8th*** day of age.
2. Hinny is a cross of male ***horse.***
3. The swine has ***38*** chromosomes.
4. Sheds for pig are known as ***sties.***
5. Dhaman heat occurs ***9th*** day after foaling.
6. Camel has biannulate ***T*** shaped uterus.
7. Average age of puberty in filly is ***12-15*** months.
8. Single humped camel is called as ***dromedary.***
9. Goat has ***60*** chromosomes.
10. ***Dolly*** breed of sheep was created by electro fusion of diploid nucleus.
11. Jamnapari breed of goat is a ***dual*** purpose breed.
12. Shearing can be done ***twice*** per year.
13. Pregnancy period of goat is ***145-150*** days.
14. Length of oestrous cycle in goat is ***17-20*** days.
15. Ganjam breed belongs to ***Orissa*** state.
16. The floor space requirement of adult goat is ***1.25-1.5 sq.m.***
17. There are two species of domestic camel viz. ***Camelus dromedarius and Camelus bactrianus***.
18. The ears of horses of ***Kathiawari*** breed tend to meet each other at the tips.
19. ***Haemolytic*** test should be done before suckling the newly born foals.
20. The pigs of large white Yorkshire breed have ***erect*** ears and ***coiled*** tail.

21. Breeding the mare in ***foaling heat*** is a common practice at large equine farm.

22. The air space per horse provided in stables is ***1296 cubic feet.***

23. The zoological name of domestic yak is ***Bos grunniens.***

24. Irregular setting of hair coat in horses is called ***whorls.***

25. ***Keratin*** gives wool the non inflammable property.

26. In India, stocking density is ***more*** than the carrying capacity of common grazing lands.

27. Fibre diameter of the carpet wool should be ***29 to 34*** microns.

28. One hank of yarn is about ***511.8*** meters in length.

29. The spinning count system was developed in ***U.K.***

30. Machine shearing leaves about ***0.48*** cams of wool on the body of sheep.

31. A narrow path with gates used for sorting sheep in groups is called ***cutting to chute.***

32. India ranks ***2nd*** in goat population in the world.

33. Process of regression of uterus from pregnant to nonpregnant state is called ***involution.***

34. Main equipment used for handling the camel consists of a ***nose peg*** and a ***nose rope.***

35. The practice of self-feeding of concentrates to young pigs in a separate enclosure away from their dams is known as ***creep feeding.***

36. The camels, according to their suitability for a particular work, have been broadly divided in to three categories, namely ***baggage camel***, ***ridding camel*** and ***draught camel.***

37. Shoeing in horse should be done by an experienced ***ferrier.***

38. The horse should clean up its feed in about ***30 minutes***.

39. A sexually matured male camel may serve upto ***50 or 60*** she camels during single breeding season.

40. Dressing percent of swine vary from 60 to ***70*** percent.

41. There are ***40*** breeds of sheep and ***20*** breeds of goat in India.

42. The occurrence of first heat period is usually regarded as an indication of ***puberty.***

43. Wool production is largely dependent upon the fleece weight and ***staple length.***

44. Name the two breeds of goat famous for pashmina ***Chegu and Changthangi.***

45. Indian sheep are usually shorn twice a year i.e. during ***March*** and in ***September***.

46. Sheep in India are reared under two different systems ***migratory*** and ***stationary.***

47. Most common symptoms of external parasitism are ***itching*** and losses of ***patches*** of wool.

48. Breeding bucks and does in advance stage of pregnancy or lactation are fed an additional ***200 to 300*** g of concentrate each day.

49. Pashmina is obtained from ***north temperate*** region of India.

50. ***Rajasthan*** state of India produces highest quantity of wool.

51. The habitat of jamanapari is ***Agra*** district.

52. The chromosomes number of goat is ***60.***

53. Castrated male sheep is known as ***either.***

54. The golden footed sheep is known as ***Merino.***

55. Fine wool contains ***25-30*** crimps per inch.

56. Feeding habit of goat is known as ***browsing.***

57. The scientific name of Indian wild boar is ***Susscrofa cristatus.***

58. The chromosome number in horse and ass is ***64 and 62,*** respectively.

59. The horses consume ***25 to 50*** liters of water per day.

60. Pre starter ration is given to piglets when they are ***2 week*** old.

61. The stallion requires ***1-4*** hours of exercise daily.

62. Jhooling is a disease commonly seen in ***camel*** species.

63. Training of camel should be practiced between the ages of ***2½ to 3 years.***

64. The boar generally reaches puberty at the age of ***8*** months.

65. Sheep belongs to the family ***bovidae.***

66. A ram can be used for breeding at the age of ***7-8 months***.

67. A ram of 2 to 2½ year_age is sufficient for ***30 to 40*** numbers of ewes.
68. Docking is generally performed when the age of lamb is ***10*** days.
69. Castration in sheep is performed at ***3 weeks*** age.
70. Sheep can be sheared ***twice*** in a year.
71. Goat can get ***80%*** of its nutritive requirement through browsing.
72. The home tract of Marwari breed of horse is ***Rajasthan.***
73. Yak milk contains ***7.3%*** butter fat.
74. Gestation period of camel is ***12 months.***
75. The first heat after foaling is termed as ***foal heat.***
76. Piglets should be weaned at ***56 days*** of age.
77. Middle Yorkshire is a product of ***large white X small white.***
78. The best age to train a camel for riding is ***one*** years.
79. The hair over the crest is called ***mane.***
80. Pashmina is obtained from ***goat.***
81. ***African boar*** is an African goat breed popularly used for upgrading the native breeds for meat purpose.
82. The method of tying the goats with rope is known as ***tethering.***
83. The example of fodder trees are ***subabool/dasrath/ker/peepal/neem.***
84. Sheep require ***sulphur*** containing amino acids for growth of wool fiber.
85. Before breeding season starts, wool around the penile region should be clipped, this process is termed as ***ringing.***
86. If cutting of hairs is known as clipping then clipping of wool is ***shearing.***
87. The goat breed named ***Nubian*** is supposed to have originated from a city of East Africa.
88. For breeding purpose, ***30 to 40 mares*** can be allotted to stallion.
89. Tamworth breed derives its name from the town of ***Tamworth*** in U.K.
90. The boar reaches puberty at the age of ***8 months.***
91. Ponies stand less than ***1.47*** meter in height.
92. The trot is a pace of ***2*** times.

93. Foals are weaned at the age of ***6*** months.
94. Large White Yorkshire is a native breed of ***U.K.***
95. Rambouillet has been crossed with Malpura to evolve ***Avikalin*** breed of sheep.
96. Rambouillet is one of the ***fine*** wool breeds.
97. Barbari breed of goat originated from ***Barbara*** area of South Africa.
98. ***Chokla*** breed produces the finest wool among the Rajasthan breeds.
99. ***Nellore*** is the tallest breed of sheep in India.
100. ***Jamnapari*** breed of goat has parrot mouth appearance.
101. Avivastra is evolved by crossing ***Chokla and Nali*** with Rambouillet and Merino breed.

10

Livestock Production & Management (PART-III)Avian, Lab, Pet, Wild & Zoo Animal Care and Management

Q.1. True or False

1.	True	Capon is a castrated male chicken.
2.	True	Pea comb is present in Cornish breed of chicken.
3.	False	Birds from 8 to 20 weeks should be provided 24 hrs light.
4.	False	Maximum crude fiber level in broiler ration is 12 percent.
5.	True	Orientation of poultry shed should be in east-west direction.
6.	True	Eggs are set in the incubator with broad end up.
7.	False	Eggs are transferred to hatcher on 14th day of incubation.
8.	True	Oval shaped, medium sized eggs are selected for hatching.
9.	True	Labrador dogs are trained for detecting narcotics/explosives.
10.	False	Rabbit has tendency of attacking from hind legs.
11.	True	The newly born guinea pig starts eating soon after birth.
12.	False	Never plug the ears with cotton wool when a dog is bathed.
13.	True	Time of mating a female dog is after stoppage of blood discharge.
14.	False	English Angora is famous for silky wool.
15.	True	White tiger is the recessive mutant of an Indian race.
16.	True	Only the adult female musk deer is hunted for musk.

17.	True	Asian elephants are grazers while African elephants are browsers.
18.	True	Yaks have low mortality rate.
19.	True	Birds of prey are called falcons.
20.	True	Poultry refers to all domestic birds that are commercially useful to man.
21.	True	The male duck is called drake.
22.	True	The mediterranean class of poultry has white ear lobe.
23.	True	Rabbits are born hairless with eyes closed.
24.	True	The tail of rat is thicker and serrated.
25.	False	Gall bladder is present in hamster.
26.	False	In rabbit, mating is allowed only in the female cage.
27.	True	Provide training to the pet dog within an hour of feeding.
28.	True	Main meal to adult dog should be given in late afternoon.
29.	True	Indian birds of prey are called raptor.
30.	False	The ovulation is spontaneous in tigress.
31.	True	Catla is a surface feeder.
32.	True	Black buck is the only Indian antelope in India.
33.	True	Duck is known as living manuring machine in fish pond.
34.	True	Grass carp feeds on weeds in pond.
35.	False	Smaller breed of poultry has a lower body temperature than larger breeds.
36.	False	Usually early moulters are good layers.
37.	True	Aseel is an Indian breed.
38.	False	Decreasing the humidity of the setter lengthens the incubation period.
39.	True	RIR is a dual purpose breed.
40.	False	All chickens have colour vision.
41.	False	Heavy breeds are very good layers.

42.	False	Incidence of broken eggs are much more in the layers kept on litter floor.
43.	True	Rats, rabbits, guinea pigs, apes etc. are used for research probably because of their genomic similarities with human beings.
44.	False	Rabbits are not herbivorous.
45.	True	Rabbits show induced ovulation.
46.	True	Neuter is the castrated feline male.
47.	False	Farrowing of rabbit occurs ones in a year.
48.	False	Greyhound is a non-sporting breed of dog.
49.	True	Rabbits are highly prolific.
50.	True	Doberman and Labrador are easy dogs to train.
51.	True	Deer and antelope are natural members of the wild life community.
52.	False	Corbet National Park is situated in Uttar Pradesh.
53.	False	Tortoise does not require vitamin and minerals.
54.	True	Salamander is an amphibian.
55.	True	Spotted deer is also known as cheetal.
56.	True	Panda is the name given to Chinese bear.
57.	True	Chemical restraint of animals is one of the most modern and best methods for dealing large and ferocious species.
58.	True	Antelopes have permanent horns.
59.	True	Rooster is the term given to an adult male chicken.
60.	False	When the egg is first laid it contains small air cell.
61.	True	Beak trimming helps to prevent cannibalism in the flock.
62.	True	The critical periods for embryonic mortality are first 2 to 4 days and 19-21 days of incubation.
63.	False	Curled toe paralysis is caused by manganese deficiency.
64.	True	First candling is done to eliminate the infertile eggs.
65.	False	The process of selecting productive birds is called culling.

66.	True	Sexual maturity occurs in chickens at about 22-24 weeks of age.
67.	True	Water requirement of rabbit depends on the climate, activity and size of the rabbit.
68.	False	Whitten effect is much more marked in rats than in mouse.
69.	True	Corprophagy in rabbit helps in recycling of undigested food in the droopings.
70.	False	Natural mating is accomplished by taking buck to the hutch of doe and never vice versa.
71.	True	Puppies start eating solid food at about 3 weeks of age and can be separated from the bitch at 6 weeks.
72.	True	Five or six days before kindling, the nest box is placed in the cage with does.
73.	True	Bunnies are born with their eyes shut and without fur.
74.	True	The crude protein content of the diets of guinea-pig should vary between 10-20 percent.
75.	True	Monkeys are highly susceptible to tuberculosis.
76.	True	Majority of the amphibians are oviparous.
77.	False	Fish in which eggs hatch internally and the young receive nourishment from mother before extrusion are called oviparous.
78.	False	Fishes of different sea depth do not differ in their morphological characteristics.
79.	False	In our elephants both male and female carry tusks.
80.	True	Most important single physical factor affecting trout hatching success is the water supply.
81.	True	Elephants are the largest terrestrial mammals presently inhabiting the earth.
82.	True	Reptiles are considered to be cold blooded animals.
83.	True	Eggs selected for hatching should be uniform in size, shape, weight and colour.
84.	False	Eggs of large size (above 60 g) show better hatchability.

85.	*True*	*Brooders should provide chicks with a wide range of temperatures.*
86.	*False*	*Egg production and egg size are not dependent on protein content of the diet.*
87.	*False*	*The act of laying eggs in hen is termed as ovulation.*
88.	*True*	*Laying hens are seldom kept in the flock beyond 19 months of age.*
89.	*True*	*Incubation in birds corresponds to gestation in domestic farm animals.*
90.	*False*	*Broiler female chick less than 5 weeks of age is called pullet.*
91.	*True*	*Puppies are born with their eyes and ears closed.*
92.	*True*	*Rabbits are characterized by the process of induced ovulation.*
93.	*False*	*Guinea pigs are more susceptible to cold than heat under tropical conditions.*
94.	*True*	*One can increase the survival rate by synchronizing kindling, thereby making room for roistering the young ones.*
95.	*True*	*For the first 20 days, baby rabbit's only food is their mother's milk.*
96.	*True*	*Harem system is one in which the males and females are run together, but separated prior to parturition.*
97.	*True*	*Digestibility of cereal diet is improved in dog by cooking.*
98.	*False*	*Guinea-pigs are naturally omnivorous in nature in the wild.*
99.	*True*	*In fishes, fungal, protozoal and trematodal infection can often be controlled with chemical bath.*
100.	*True*	*At all stages reptiles breathe air by means of lungs.*
101.	*True*	*Identification method in fish which causes less damage is hot or cold branding.*
102.	*True*	*Certain type of weeds in water bodies can be controlled by means of selected varieties of herbivorous fish like grass carp.*
103.	*False*	*The food consumed by elephant in wild is low in fibre.*

104. True *Before selecting a suitable site for collection of spawn, a* survey is conducted for topography, distribution and composition of fish fauna.

105. False Specific type of ponds is not required for the culture of particular species of fish and their life history stages.

106. True Induced breeding is carried out by hypothalamus extract injection for breeding of carps for seed production.

107. True Project tiger was started in 1973 in India.

108. True The common carp is a universal donor.

109. False WWF (India) was set up in 1961.

110. True The cross breed male yak is always sterile.

111. True Catla breeds in rivers during rainy season.

112. False Wild life Protection Act has ten schedules.

113. True Lime is necessary to increase pH of water in fish ponds.

114. True Phosphoric acid is the initiator of rigor mortis in fish meat.

115. True Mating of rabbits are allowed only in the male cages.

116. True Tail of mice is thinner and not serrated.

117. True Plug the ears with cotton wool when the dogs are bathed.

118. True Hamster suffers mostly from wet tail infections.

119. False Debeaking is done at 6 months of age.

120. False Pause is the number of days the birds laid eggs.

121. False Provide 24 hrs light to birds from 8-20 weeks of age.

122. True White Pekin and Muscovy are the meat producing breeds of duck.

123. True Aspergillosis in birds is commonly known as brooder pneumonia.

124. False Temperature of brooder house should be reduced by 7^0C every successive week till it reaches 21^0C.

125. False The incubation period of quail is 31 days.

126. True Forced moulting is also known as recycling.

127. True — BBLW stand for broad breasted large white.

128. True — Preovipositional death takes place because of chromosomal abnormalities.

129. True — Pomeranian is a non-sporting breed of dog.

130. False — The daily intake of solid food in growing pups after weaning would be approximately 15 percent of its body weight.

131. False — In female dog gestation period is 120 days.

132. True — In rabbit breeding is very fast with gestation period of about 31 days.

133. False — Hamster is a short squat rodent without tail.

134. True — Tyzzer's disease affects mice as well as other lab animal also.

135. True — Rabbit meat containing low fat and cholesterol is categorized as pearly white colour meat.

136. True — Gnotobiotic animal are breed in controlled environment.

137. True — In fish, breeding and spawning can be induced by HCG and crude pituitary extract.

138. True — Copper sulphate is the chemical of choice for controlling algal bloom.

139. True — Rhinoceros defecate at particular spot.

140. True — Nembutal is an immobilizing agent.

141. True — Reptiles are poikilothermic.

142. False — Shotgun and projectile rifles are most commonly used in the field condition for restraining small wild animals.

143. False — Wild life protection act was enacted by Government of India in year 1982.

144. False — IFAW stands for Indian Fund for Animal Welfare.

Q.2. Multiple Choice Questions :

1. White Leghorn belongs to the :

   a. English class **b. Mediterranean class**

   c. American class d. None of the above

2. Best time for first candling of eggs after setting is:

a. 1st day **b. 4th to 5th day**

c. 18th day d. None of the above

3. In chicks the brooding temperature in first week should be:

a. 45°C **b. 35°C**

c. 25°C d. None of the above

4. Optimum temperature for incubation of chicken egg is:

a. 34.5°C **b. 37.5°C**

c. 40.5°C d. None of the above

5. The site of fertilization of egg in a poultry is:

a. Infundibulum b. Magnum

c. Isthmus d. None of the above

6. In poultry birds the functional organ is only:

a. Left ovary b. Right ovary

c. Both ovaries d. None of the above

7. The incubation period of chicken egg is:

a. 21days b. 28 days

c. 35 days d. None of the above

8. The best meat breed of duck is:

a. Indian Runner **b. White Pekin**

c. Khaki Campbell d. None of the above

9. Cannibalism is more pronounced in:

a. Hamster b. Rat

c. Mice d. None of the above

10. Docking in pet dogs after birth is done on:

a. 5-10th day b. 20-25th day

c. 40-45th day d. None of the above

11. The gestation period of rabbit is:

a. 30-32 days b. 21-22 days

c. 16-18 days d. None of the above

12. The laboratory animal which has check pouches:

a. Mice **b. Hamster**

c. Guinea pig d. None of the above

13. At present largest angora wool producing state is:

a. Himachal Pradesh b. Haryana

c. Rajasthan d. None of the above

14. The market age of rabbit is:

a. 3 months b. 6 months

c. 9 months d. None of the above

15. Gestation period of cat is:

a. 30-32 days **b. 60-65 days**

c. 90-95 days d. None of the above

16. The scientific name of Asian elephant is:

a. Elephas maximus b. Loxodonta africana

c. Both of the above d. None of the above

17. The dissolved oxygen in fish pond water should be:

a. > 4mg/L b. < 4 mg/L

c. Both of the above d. None of the above

18. For maximum fish production, ratio of Catla: Rohu: Mrigal to be stocked in ponds should be:

a. 10:30:70 **b. 30:40:30**

c. 50:40:10 d. None of the above

19. WWF (International) launched in the year:

a. 1951 **b. 1961**

c. 1971 d. None of the above

20. Bear belong to the family:
    a. Pongidae **b. Ursidae**
    c. Procyonidae d. None of the above
21. WWF (India) was launched in the year:
    a. 1949 b. 1959
    c. 1969 d. None of the above
22. The status of tiger in India is:
    a. Threatened **b. Endangered**
    b. Vulnerable c. None of the above
23. The Kanha National Park is located in:
    a. U.P. b. Uttarakhand
    c. M.P. d. None of the above
24. The incubation temperature for chicken egg is:
    a. 34.2-35.5^{0}C **b. 37.2–37.5^{0}C**
    c. 38.5-39.5^{0}C d. None of the above
25. Good layers have moulting:
    a. Late & slowly **b. Early & rapid**
    c. Early & slowly d. None of the above
26. The complete formation of egg requires:
    a. 18-20 hrs **b. 24-26 hrs**
    c. 30-32 hrs d. None of the above
27. Popular breed of Indian game fowl is:
    a. Aseel b. Cornis
    c. Kadaknath d. None of the above
28. The type of comb in White Leghorn is:
    a. Pea b. Rose
    c. Single d. None of the above

29. Male chicken between 18 weeks to one year of age is called:

    a. Cockerel b. Broiler

    c. Capon d. None of the above

30. During debeaking, which portion of beak is removed:

    a. Lower beak **b. Upper beak**

    c. Both a & b d. None of the above

31. The gestation period in rat is:

    a. 16-18 days **b. 21 days**

    c. 30-32 days d. None of the above

32. Laboratory animal which are used for cancer tissue testing is:

    a. Guinea pigs **b. Hamsters**

    c. Rats d. None of the above

33. Among lab animals, cannibalism is more pronounced in:

    a. Hamster **b. Mice**

    c. Rat d. None of the above

34. The lab animal use for toxicological studies is:

    a. Rabbit b. Mice

    c. Hamster d. None of the above

35. Vitamin C feeding is essential in:

    a. Guinea pig b. Rabbit

    c. Mice d. None of the above

36. Ovulation occurs at the time of copulation in:

    a. Rabbit b. Rat

    c. Mice d. None of the above

37. Dogs trained to detect narcotics and explosives are:

    a. Pomeranian **b. Labradors**

    c. Alsatian d. None of the above

38. Indian wild life (protection) Act came into existence in year:

a. 1952 | b. 1069

c. 1972 | d. None of the above

39. The area for national parks and sanctuaries recommended by the expert committee is:

a. 25 percent | b. 8 percent

c. 4 percent | d. None of the above

40. Deer belongs to the family:

a. Cervidae | b. Felidae

c. Moschidae | d. None of the above

41. Bear belongs to the family:

a. Ursidae | b. Pongidae

c. Procyonidae | d. None of the above

42. The ideal pH for fish pond water should be:

a. 4.0 – 4.5 | b. 6.0 – 6.5

c. 7.5 – 8.5 | d. None of the above

43. The flagship wild species in India is:

a. Tiger | b. Black buck

c. Peacock | d. None of the above

44. Mediterranean breeds of poultry includes:

a. White Plymouth Rock | b. Rhode Island Red

c. White Leghorn | d. White Cornish

45. Ranikhet disease is caused by:

a. Bacteria | b. Parasite

c. Virus | d. Nutritional deficiency

46. The best method of pedigree hatching is:

a. Flock mating | **b. Pen mating**

c. Shift mating | d. Stud mating

47. The shells or weak bones of layers require attention to adjust the level of:

a. Calcium
b. Phosphorous
c. Vitamin D
d. All of the above

48. Persistent layer moult:

a. Late and rapid
b. Late and slowly
c. Early and slowly
d. Early and rapidly

49. The number of eggs a hen will lay during a year depends upon:

a. Age at sexual maturity
b. Persistency
c. intensity of lay
d. All of the above

50. Factors necessary for successful incubation includes:

a. Temperature
b. Humidity
c. Turning of eggs
d. All of the above

51. Identification of rabbit can be done by:

a. Leg banding
b. Ear banding
c. Tattooing
d. All of the above

52. The breed of rabbit include:

a. Gray giant
b. Great dane
c. Persian
d. Tabby

53. It is necessary to deworm dog after every:

a. Three years
b. Three months
c. Three weeks
d. Three days

54. Toy breeds of dog are preferred:

a. For hunting
b. As guards
c. As companions
d. All of the above

55. Which of the following laboratory animal is used for immunological studies:

a. Rat
b. Mice
c. Rabbit
d. Guinea pig

56. Selection of a broiler rabbit depends upon:

a. Breed
b. Feed conversion ratio
c. Kidding percentage
d. All of the above

57. Docking is carried out at the age of:

a. 4-10 days
b. 4-10 weeks
c. 4-10 months
d. 1-2 years

58. In dog heat remains for:

a. 10-12 hours
b. 3-8 hours
c. 10-12 days
d. 2-5 days

59. The zoos are established for:

a. Recreation
b. Conservation
c. Research
d. All of the above

60. Kaziranga National Park has been created specially to protect:

a. Asiatic lion
b. Rhinoceros
c. Tiger
d. Panther

61. A comprehensive central legislation called the wildlife act was enacted in the year:

a. 1972
b. 1982
c. 1992
d. 2002

62. Asiatic lion is found in:

a. Gir National park
b. Kanha National park
c. Corbet National park
d. Dudhwa National park

63. Nilgai is a:

a. Antelope
b. Deer
c. Musk deer
d. Rhinoceros

64. Larger animals which are widely spread in the rain forests include:

a. Sambhar deer
b. Wild boar
c. Elephant
d. All of the above

65. Dudhwa National Park is located in:

a. Nainital b. Bareilly

c. Lakhimpur Kheri d. Agra

66. The average age of elephant is :

a. 40 years **b. 60 years**

c. 80 years d. 100 years

67. During the first week of brooding, temperature inside the brooder houses is maintained at:

a. 100^0 F **b. 95^0 F**

c. 90^0 F d. 85^0 F

68. Random sample test for layers and broilers provides valuable information about:

a. Ranking of different genetic stocks

b. Commercial viability of the stock

c. Genetic progress achieved in their performance over time

d. All of the above

69. How many times hatching eggs should be turned in 24 hours in a setter:

a. Two times **b. Six times**

c. Eight times d. Twelve times

70. For good hatchability eggs selected should be:

a. Above 60 gm b. 45 to 50 gm

c. 50 to 55 gm d. 55 to 60 gm

71. Laying and breeding hens normally require protein in their diet at levels (percent):

a. 18 **b. 15**

c. 12 d. 24

72. Piperazine compounds are commonly used in poultry against infections:

a. Bacteria **b. Worm**

c. Viral d. Fungal

73. Housing space requirement per adult hen is:

a. 3 sq. ft.
b. 3.5 sq ft.
c. 2.0 sq ft.
d. 1.5 sq. ft.

74. The organism transmitted through eggs that affects hatchability directly is:

a. E.coli
b. Pullorum
c. Spirochaetes
d. All the above

75. The optimum percentage of crude fibre in the diet of rabbit is:

a. 5 to 10
b. 10 to 15
c. 15 to 20
d. 20 to 25

76. The average litter size of rabbit is:

a. 1-3
b. 6-10
c. 11-14
d. 3-5

77. Gestation period of dog is :

a. 50-60 days
b. 60-65 days
c. 65-70 days
d. 70-75 days

78. The floor space required by a rabbit weighing approximately 2 kg is:

a. 1.00 sq.m.
b. 0.90 sq.m.
c. 0.14 sq.m.
d. 1.40 sq.m.

79. The estrus cycle in rabbit is:

a. No estrus cycle
b. 20-22 days
c. 28-29 days
d. 8-12 days

80. When one or more males are housed with several females, the breeding system is referred as:

a. Monogamy
b. Hand mating
c. Polygamy
d. Harem system

81. Proper steps of housing of rabbit include:

a. High state of cleanliness
b. Dry and well ventilated
c. Vermin proof doors
d. All of the above

82. Age at fertile making in male guinea-pig is:

a. 30-35 days
b. 60-80 days
c. 100-120 days
d. Above 150 days

83. Based upon the feeding strategies, reptiles can be categorized as either:

a. Herbivorous
b. Omnivorous
c. Carnivorous
d. All of the above

84. There were only a few indigenous fish prior to the introduction of exotic fishes which was:

a. Golden carp
b. Grass carp
c. Mahseer
d. English carp

85. Before selecting a suitable site for collection of spawn, a survey is conducted for ascertaining:

a. Topography
b. Distribution and composition of fish farm
c. Accessibility of the site
d. All of the above

86. Fish production is influenced substantially by:

a. Water temperature
b. Oxygen content of water
c. The amount of food produced or fed
d. All of the above

87. Monkeys are normally given the feed in which of the following form:

a. Coarsely ground feed
b. Pellets
c. Wafers
d. Whole grains

88. During incubation of fish egg, the egg passes through several stages which are:

a. Green egg and eyed egg
b. Sac fry and swim up fry
c. Both a & b
d. None of the above

89. Amphibians are commonly used in laboratories to acquaint the beginning biology students:

a. Main features of vertebrates anatomy

b. To study physiology

c. Providing abundant embryonic material

d. All of the above

90. The handling of snake present a special problem because of the:

a. Wide spread fear of them

b. An elongated shape

c. Vermonous nature of certain kind

d. All of the above

91. The optimum temperature for hatching eggs in the incubator is between:

a. 98.6^{0}F to 100.4^{0}F b. 100^{0}F to 101^{0}F

c. 100^{0}F to 110^{0}F d. 96^{0}F to 98^{0}F

92. The incubated eggs should be candled on:

a. 3rd or 4th day **b. 7th or 8th day**

c. 12th or 13 day d. 16th or 18th day

93. What should be the maximum limit of crude fibre in the preparation of poultry mash:

a. 4 percent **b. 7 percent**

c. 10 percent d. 15 percent

94. A poultry house may be:

a. Economical b. Durable

c. Provide comfort and safety **d. All of the above**

95. It is well established that chicken need vitamin A at:

a. Chicken stage b. Grower stage

c. Layer stage **d. All of the above**

96. Chicken are vaccinated against Marek's disease:

a. On the 21 day after hatch b. On the 4th day after hatch

c. Immediately after hatch d. All of the above

97. The floor space in layer birds depend upon:

a. Type of floor
b. Size of bird
c. Temperature and ventilation
d. All of the above

98. Feed conversion of layers in influenced by:

a. Metabolisable energy content of the diet.
b. Pen temperature
c. Rate of egg production
d. All of the above

99. The site of fermentation of crude fibre in rabbits is:

a. Large intestine
b. Small intestine
c. Caecum
d. Colon

100. Whelping is the act of giving birth in:

a. Rabbit
b. Cat
c. Dog
d. Rat

101. The best method of identification of guinea pig is:

a. Ear marking
b. Ear clips
c. Staining
d. Natural coat colour

102. The cages of rats and mice are in general solids from sides with:

a. Perforated top
b. Perforated floor
c. Both of the above
d. None of the above

103. Average litter size of rat is:

a. 10-12
b. 6-10
c. 2-4
d. 1-4

104. The surface area requirement for adult mouse is:

a. 10 sq. cm.
b. 100 sq. cm.
c. 1000 sq. cm.
d. 1 sq. cm.

105. Comfort zone of temperature in modern animal house is:

a. 10-15^{0}C
b. 15-18^{0}C
c. 20-21^{0}C
d. 25-30^{0}C

106. The major causes of mortality during transporting seedling or small fishes is due to:

a. Low oxygen b. High carbon dioxide

c. High oxygen d. Low carbon dioxide

107. The number of fish to stock in a pond is related to:

a. Its surface area b. The level of food production

c. The size of fish desired **d. All of the above**

108. Selective breeding in fishes has achieved spectacular increase in the rate of:

a. Growth

b. Number of eggs per female

c. Egg size

d. All of the above

109. A useful strategy for formulating diets for captive wild animal is to consider:

a. Dietary habits in the wild

b. Oral and gastro morphology

c. Cage and enclosure environment

d. All of the above

110. For a successful fish farming the temperature of lake or reservoir should be about:

a. 0^0C b. 10^0C

c. 20^0C d. 30^0C

111. Elephants spend most of their time in:

a. Feeding b. Bathing

c. Drinking **d. All of the above**

112. Handling, restraint and immobilization of wild animals is of paramount importance for their:

a. Capture b. Clinical examination

c. Administration of medicines **d. All of the above**

113. Name the vertebrates which require both terrestrial as well as aquatic habitats to complete life cycle:

a.	Reptiles	**b.**	**Amphibian**
c.	Primates	d.	Carnivores

114. The wild life expert committee recommended area for national park and sanctuaries in India:

a.	**4 percent**	b.	10 percent
c.	8 percent	d.	None of the above

115. The first zoo in India was set up in year:

a.	**1859**	b.	1954
c.	1974	d.	None of the above

116. Musk deer belongs to the family:

a.	Carvidae	**b.**	**Moschidae**
c.	Ursidae	d.	None of the above

117. One rabbit buck for breeding is kept for how many number of does:

a.	**10-12**	b.	20-24
c.	30-36	d.	None of the above

118. In first week, the brooding temperature should be:

a.	45^0C	**b.**	**35^0C**
c.	25^0C	d.	None of the above

119. According to nutritional advisory committee, the average Indian diet should contain:

a.	100 eggs/person/year	b.	250 eggs/person/year
c.	**180 eggs/person/year**	d.	400 eggs/person/year

120. Which of the following is a game bird of India and famous for its fighting ability:

a.	Nacked neck	**b.**	**Aseel**
c.	White Cornish	d.	None of the above

121. Wyandotte breed of poultry belong to which of the following class:

a. American b. English

c. Mediterranean d. Both b & c

122. Khaki Campbell is the cross bred duck developed in which of the following Country:

a. India **b. England**

c. Australia d. None of the above

123. Infectious coryza is a respiratory disease of adult and growing bird caused by:

a. Staphylococcus aureus b. Mycoplasma gallisepticum

c. Haemophilus gallinarum d. Protozoa

124. In brooder house the most comfortable temperature during first week should be:

a. 32^0- 35^0C b. 10^0-15^0C

c. 5^0-10^0C d. None of the above

125. Earthen pitcher and Kunnali equipment in poultry house mainly serve the purpose for:

a. Feeding b. Debarking

c. Watering d. Brooding

126. Floor space requirement for light breed bird at 9-12 week of age is:

a. 100 cm^2/bird b. 450 cm^2/bird

c. 950 cm^2/ bird d. 1600 cm^2/bird

127. New Zealand White breed is an example of:

a. Meat breed b. Wool breed

c. Angora breed d. None of the above

128. A lactating female rabbit while nursing should consume concentrate mixture on an average:

a. 100 g/day b. 1kg/day

c. 1.5 kg/day **d. 250 g/day**

129. Act of parturition in bitch is known as:

a.	**Whelping**	b.	Kidding
c.	Farrowing	d.	Both b & c

130. Shearing should be planned in rabbit when the wool length is:

a.	25 cm	**b.**	**6 cm**
c.	2 cm	d.	20 cm

131. The dog breed with short hair, feathered tail and body covered with long hair falling on eyes:

a.	Bull mastiff	b.	Australian terrier
c.	Grey hound	**d.**	**Lhasa apso**

132. The command in dog training to identify the object through its strong power of smell is commonly known as:

a.	Carry	b.	Fetch
c.	Do not touch	**d.**	**Retrieve**

133. SPF stands for:

a.	**Specific pathogen free**	b.	Special pathological form
c.	Specific pathognomic form	d.	None of the above

134. Puberty appears in dog at age of:

a.	10-15 month	**b.**	**20-24 month**
c.	4 years	d.	5 years

135. Lions live in groups are called:

a.	Pack	b.	Herd
c.	**Pride**	d.	None of the above

136. Which of the following is an immobilization emergency:

a.	Bloat	b.	Respiratory arrest
c.	Shock	**d.**	**All of the above**

137. Feline panleucopenia is a highly contagious disease of felidae family caused by:

a.	Mycobacterium	b.	Rhabdovirus
c.	**Parvovirus**	d.	All of the above

138. Gestation period of elephant is:

a.	310 days	b.	250 days
c.	150 days	**d.**	**630 days**

Q.3. Fill up the Blanks :

1. Broad end of the egg is kept on the ***upper*** side during storage of eggs.
2. During incubation period turning of eggs is done at an interval of ***4-6*** hrs.
3. ***Fish meal*** is a source of animal protein in the poultry ration.
4. Under intensive deep litter system per layer floor space provided is ***2.5-3.0*** sq.ft.
5. The maximum level of crude fibre in layer ration is ***10.5 %.***
6. The toy breeds of dog are popularly called as ***lady lap*** dogs.
7. Cats are sensitive to ***streptomycin*** drug by any route.
8. Judging of dogs is based on the breed and obedience.
9. Training is easier in dogs of ***Doberman/Alsatian*** breed.
10. In female dog, heat period lasts for ***10-12*** days.
11. Never put hand to touch ***head and nostril*** of a dog.
12. ***Hamster*** is a lab animal used for testing of cancer tissue.
13. ***Mayana*** is a popular singing and talking pet bird.
14. The rutting call of yak is called as ***mutus.***
15. Flehman's behaviour is common in ***barasingha.***
16. The scientific name of Asian elephant is ***Elephas maximus.***
17. The wild life act has ***6*** chapters and ***5*** schedules.
18. ***H. Gibbon*** is the only ape found in India.
19. RIR is ***dual*** purpose breed.
20. Kadaknath breed of poultry originated from ***Jhabua/Dhar*** (M.P.).
21. Dressing percentage in cockerel is ***less*** while in broiler it is ***73 percent.***
22. Egg white and egg shell of an egg is formed in ***magnum and uterus.***
23. Egg producing breed of poultry are ***Leghorn*** and ***Anconas.***

24. As per recommendation of ICMR, one must consume ***180*** eggs in a year.
25. The diet recommended as per NRC for guinea pig should have ***18 %*** CP and ***136*** kcal mE.
26. Cannibalism is more in ***hamster*** animal.
27. Rats are ***laboratory*** animal.
28. Mice require ***65-70⁰F*** temperature and ***40-70 %*** humidity.
29. Weaning in rabbits is done between ***5 to 6*** weeks.
30. Optimum temperature in the laying shed for maximum production should be ***55-65⁰F.***
31. The distance between pubic bones in good layers should be ***2-3*** fingers distance.
32. No turning of eggs is required after ***18 days*** of incubation.
33. The best egg laying variety of chicken is ***White Leghorn.***
34. The brooding temperature in the first week for chicks should be ***35⁰C.***
35. Chicks should be given ***24 hrs*** light including day light.
36. Rabbit meat has ***low*** cholesterol level.
37. One rabbit buck is kept for ***8-10*** numbers of does.
38. The gestation period in rabbit is ***30-33*** days.
39. Pregnancy in hamster is diagnosed with the presence of ***mucosal plug.***
40. Among all lab animals ***hamster*** is free from serious infections.
41. Rabbit mature at the age of ***6-8*** months.
42. The scientific name of tiger is ***Panthera tigris.***
43. The musk is secreted from ***male*** musk deer.
44. Wild life protection act has ***5*** *s*chedules and ***6*** sections.
45. ***Spotted*** *deer* is the most favoured prey for tigers.
46. Indian board of wild life was constituted in the year ***1952.***
47. Project tiger was established in India in ***1973.***
48. There are two types of snake venom viz. ***neurotoxin and hemotoxin.***
49. Rutting call given by barasingha is called ***bugle.***

50. During first week of brooding most comfortable temperature (F) is ***95°F.***
51. The average egg weight of Japanese quail is ***10-13 g.***
52. In fowls egg takes about ***21*** days to hatch.
53. Clutch size is longer and inter clutch interval is shorter for the ***good*** layers.
54. A pullet is said to be ***sexually mature*** when she lays her first egg.
55. The germ spot in fertile egg is known as ***blastoderm*** whereas in infertile egg is known as ***blastodisc***.
56. Newly hatched chicks are vaccinated against ***Marek's disease (MD).***
57. Angora is ***wool*** type breed of rabbit.
58. Gestation period of rabbit is ***30-31*** days.
59. Rabbit should be fed forage in ***morning*** and concentrate in the evening.
60. Weaning period in rabbit is ***30-40*** days.
61. New Zealand ***White*** is a broiler breed of rabbit.
62. In rat and mice round worm and tick infection is due to ***mismanagement***.
63. The skin of newly born baby of rabbit is devoid of ***hair.***
64. Rabbit are efficient food converters and are highly ***prolific***.
65. Largest Indian deer is ***Sambar***.
66. Catla is a common ***fresh*** water fish.
67. Breeding of fish occurs in flooded rivers during ***monsoon*** season.
68. Average age of tiger is ***20-23*** years.
69. Antlers are found in ***deer.***
70. Tiger belongs to order ***carnivore.***
71. The deer present in Kedarnath sanctuary is ***musk deer***.
72. Gestation period of lion is ***105-106*** days.
73. Each poultry breed has several varieties which differ from one another in ***plumage, colour and combs.***
74. The ovum consists of 3 main parts namely ***vitelline membrane, cervical disc, and yolk material.***
75. Eggs are fumigated with ***formaldehyde gas***.

76. In order to get maximum laying response from the layer, the total day light should be ***14-15*** hours light/day.
77. ***Ascardia galli*** is the most common round worm of chicken.
78. The number of eggs laid by a hen on consecutive days is known as ***clutch.***
79. When baby chicks are reared successfully without any extra heat, such brooding is known as ***cold brooding.***
80. The birth of young rabbit is known as ***kindling.***
81. In dog the most reliable method of identification is by tattooing on an ear or of the abdominal wall tattooing.
82. ***February–March and August–September*** are the two common breeding periods in dogs.
83. In rabbit shearing should be done after every ***70-90*** days.
84. The protein content in the ration of growing and lactating rats is ***20*** percent.
85. In dogs normal temperature is ***102^0F,*** pulse rate ***50-112*** per minute and respiration rate ***15-25 breaths*** per minute.
86. Cat may have ***1-8*** kittens in a litter.
87. A water mold or fungus known as ***Saprolegnia*** is the most common fungus causing infection in fish.
88. In temperate and cold climates amphibian ***hibernates.***
89. Reptiles contribute a class of vertebrates that include ***snake, lizard, turtles*** and ***crocodiles.***
90. Respiratory exchange in fish is primarily a function of the ***gills.***
91. Generally elephant gives birth to only ***one*** calf.
92. In their natural habitat elephant feeds on ***root, leaves and fruits*** of various trees.
93. Fishing should begin when the fish have reached about ***75*** percent of the ponds total capacity.
94. The sense that appears to exert the greatest influence on fish behaviour is ***odour.***
95. The turkey of any sex under 16 weeks is termed as ***Frayer tester.***
96. The male duck is called ***drake.***

97. Double yoked eggs are ***unfit*** for incubation.

98. The most common method of classifying chicks has been on the basis of their origin i.e. ***American, Asiatic, English and Mediterranean.***

99. The reproductive system of male bird consists of paired testes the ***epididymis, vas deferens and penis.***

100. Removing a large portion of the comb farm day old chick is called ***dabbling***.

101. Handling, rearing and growth of chick after hatching are referred as ***brooding***.

102. Most common external parasites of chickens are ***lice and mites.***

103. Rabbits are produced for ***meat, fur wool and laboratory*** usage.

104. Rabbits are kept in cages called ***hutches*** for case of handling, protection and proper management.

105. The average age of sexual maturity of female mice is ***60*** days.

106. For the safety of the animal handler a tape muzzle should be used in ***dog***.

107. Pregnancy in dog can be detected by palpating the abdomen of the standing bitch ***21-28*** day after coitus.

108. Female dog comes in estrus for the first time between ***6 and 8*** months of age.

109. For growing, pregnant or lactating animals a level of ***25 %*** protein is recommended and for adult dog the requirement is ***10-15*** percent.

110. In dog pulse rate is recorded with the help of thumb and fingers gently pressed on ***femoral artery*** for 30 seconds or one minute.

111. Fertilization of egg is ***external*** in frog and toad.

112. Amphibians have been used for a variety of purposes, both for ***teaching and research.***

113. All snakes are ***carnivorous*** and swallow their food without chewing.

114. The simplest way to catch a snake or lizard is with a ***snake rod.***

115. ***Ammonia*** is the principal excretory product of fish and together with nitrate is very toxic.

116. The two common varieties of elephant are ***Indian and African.***

117. Full-grown elephant can consume any thing from ***270-320*** kg of green fodder a day.

118. Primates are restrained commonly by ***general, physical and chemical*** methods.

119. The national parks are established by ***legislation***.

120. Dissolved oxygen should be ***>4*** mg/litre of water for good pawning.

121. The adult musk deer is hunted for its ***musk***.

122. ***Duck*** are known as living manuring machine in a fish pond.

123. Kanha national park is located in ***Madhya Pradesh***

124. The flagship wild species in India is ***tiger.***

125. Small size breed of dogs are popularly called as ***toy dog.***

126. Mice are used for ***toxicological*** studies.

127. Removal of ovaries in female dogs is called ***spaying***.

128. Broad end of eggs is kept ***upside*** in incubator.

129. Market age of poultry broiler is ***45*** days of age.

130. Incubation period of duck egg is ***28*** days.

131. The day old chicks are given ***F_1*** and ***Marek's*** vaccination.

132. Floor space per layer in deep one litter system is ***2½-3*** sq.ft.

133. Optimum temperature in a layer house should be ***55^0 F.***

134. ***Kadaknath*** breed of poultry is a native of Jhabua and Dhar districts of M.P.

135. ***Mesovarium*** keeps ovary suspended in the body cavity.

136. ***Depigmentation*** starts from the vent in layers.

137. ***58***% of egg weight is total egg white.

138. ***Xanthophyll*** pigment is transferred from blood to yolk.

139. ***Magnum*** is a place in the oviduct of bird where all egg white proteins are secreted.

140. ***50-55*** gram is the optimum weight of chicken's egg.

141. ***70 %*** relative humidity is essential from 19-21 days during artificial incubation of chicken eggs.

142. In ***1947***, Laboratory Animal Bureau was set up in India.

143. ***60-70 %*** laboratory animals used for research purpose are mice.

144. ***Rabbit*** is also known as Cinderella of livestock.

145. ***Syrian and Chinese*** are the two popular varieties of hamster.

146. ***Avidin*** enzyme in raw egg if fed to dogs destroys vitamin biotin.

147. ***Pica*** is the condition when pet develops a tendency to eat dirt, grass, faeces etc.

148. ***Angora*** breed of rabbit is white and is reared exclusively for their excellent wool quality.

149. ***Fish meal*** is an important byproduct of fish used as a protein supplement for livestock and poultry.

150. The recommended ratio for Catla, Rohu and Mrigal in a rearing pond is ***10:20:20***

151. India ranks ***8th*** in terms of fish production.

152. ***N & P*** elements make fish meat as valuable manure.

153. The recommended ratio of salt while preserving fish by salting method is ***1:6***

154. Periyar national park and wildlife sanctuary is located in ***Kerala.***

155. ***In-situ*** method of conservation refers to the conservation of wild animal within their natural habitat.

156. ***Tigon/liger*** is the intercrossing between tiger and lion.

11

Livestock Producton and Management (PART-IV)
Cattle, Buffalo Production and Management

Q.1. True or False :

1.	True	Buffalo is a triple purpose animal.
2.	True	Cattle population is receding.
3.	True	Poll can differentiate black cow/buffalo.
4.	True	Pregnant cows must be separated two months before calving.
5.	True	Blood profiles are good index for selection.
6.	True	Frieswal is a good strain of cattle.
7.	True	Karan Fries is also a good strain of cattle.
8.	True	Tharparkar is a dual purpose breed.
9.	False	Hariana is good milch breed.
10.	True	Murrah has wedge shaped body.
11.	True	HACCP is good for quality control.
12.	True	ONBS is good for quick improvement.
13.	True	E.T.T. is favourable for better milk production.
14.	True	India is short of good bulls.
15.	False	Milk vcin is rich in milk.

16. True — Distance between teats is sign of high yielder.

17. False — The rumen in ruminants is a modified part of small intestine.

18. True — Cakes are incorporated in concentrate mixture for protein supplement.

19. False — Pregnancy supplementation is provided after 8 months of gestation in crossbred cows.

20. False — Nagpuri is the heaviest breed of buffalo.

21. True — India has about one half of the world population of buffaloes.

22. False — Bull pen should be located far away from other animals in large livestock.

23. True — The optimum group size of dairy cows for loose housing is 30-35.

24. True — The new born calf is a monogastric animal.

25. True — Trap is used for preventing back flow of sewer grasses escaping in to the house drainage systems.

26. False — Closed drainage system is ideal for cow houses.

27. True — If cow is frightened, angered or ill treated let down of milk will not occur and very little milk can be harvested.

28. True — The only method other than pedigrees available to evaluate the great bulk of dairy animal is by judging.

29. False — The area where specialized breeds already exist, crossbreeding should be permitted.

30. False — Maximum fat percent is reported in the milk of Murrah breed of buffalo.

31. True — Faster the rate of milking more the amount of milk is expected.

32. True — Feeding roughages and concentrates together in a mixed form is known as complete system of feeding.

33. True — After weaning i.e. about 3 to 4 months of age, bull calves are separated from heifer calves.

34. False — India posesses about one fifth of world cattle population.

35. False — The SNF content of milk is not influenced by high ambient temperature.

36. True Providing water spray for cows and buffaloes reduces heat stress under hot arid condition than hot humid conditions.

37. True Buffaloes are better converters of roughages into milk.

38. True Tattooing is generally done in the left ear of the calf.

39. False Humid climate is more suitable for livestock production than dry climate.

40. False Artificial induction of lactation is not possible through the use of hormone in barren cow.

41. False Silent heat is never accompanied by ovulation.

42. False Milking machine operates effectively between 150-175 inches of Hg.

43. False Pulsation ratio in machine milking is normally kept between 3:2.

44. True Bull is half of the herd.

45. False Urea feeding is recommended in young calf below 2 month of age.

46. True Heifer of 2-3 year of age is equal to 0.75 adult stock units.

47. True One person can be engaged for feeding of 25-30 calves of 0-3 month of age.

48. False Murrah is jet black coloured having tightly curved horned breed of cattle.

49. False Wide gap between wet and herd average is indication of good management.

50. False Stripping causes less irritation to teats than other methods.

51. True Tail to tail system is better than face to face system in conventional barn.

52. False Buffaloes are more heat tolerant than cattle.

53. False Dried grass or legumes stored for winter feed is termed silage.

54. True Heat period in buffaloes lasts for 18 to 36 hours.

55. True The most meaningful measurement of sex drives are the number of ejaculations and the latency of ejaculation.

56. False Animal shed should be located with long axis north to south.

57. True Out of the method of heat loss available for domestic livestock, evaporation loss is potentially most important.

58. True The calving interval in murrah buffalo is 17-18 month.

59. False Milk yield and milk constituents are not affected by decrease or increase in ambient temperature.

60. False Selection on the type alone will result in fast improvement of milk production.

61. False Quality of protein in ruminant ration is more important than non-ruminant ration.

62. True Destruction of micro organism by chemical means is called as disinfection.

63. False Head to head system of arrangement of milking cows in a two row cow house helps in reducing labour requirement.

64. False Temperate animals are in general having better heat tolerance than tropical animals.

65. False Feed stuff usually high in digestible nutrients and low in fibres are termed as roughages.

66. False Steaming up operation should be carried out in the first two month of pregnancy.

67. False A cow in heat should be inseminated between 20-24 hrs.

68. True A stall measuring 1.5m in length and 1.2m width is considered suitable for Indian cows.

69. True A substance used to kill harmful organism on non-living surfaces is called disinfectant.

70. True The average lactation yield of the Indian cow is low because of the fact that most of the breeds are draught type.

71. False Buffalo is a seasonal breeder.

72. False Legumes are good source of energy but are poor in proteins.

73. True Optimum ratio of roughage to concentrate is 60:40 for dairy cattle.

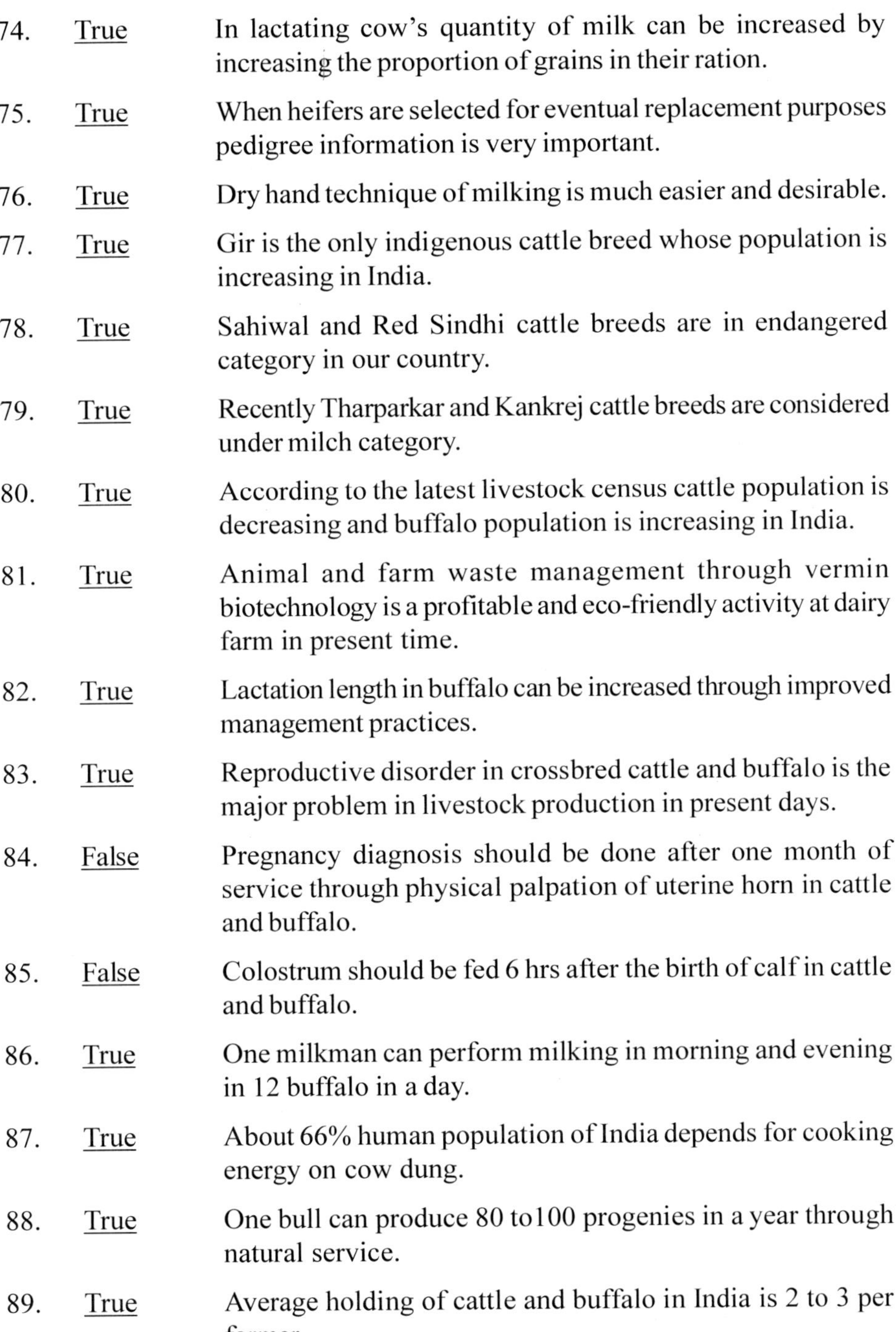

74. True In lactating cow's quantity of milk can be increased by increasing the proportion of grains in their ration.

75. True When heifers are selected for eventual replacement purposes pedigree information is very important.

76. True Dry hand technique of milking is much easier and desirable.

77. True Gir is the only indigenous cattle breed whose population is increasing in India.

78. True Sahiwal and Red Sindhi cattle breeds are in endangered category in our country.

79. True Recently Tharparkar and Kankrej cattle breeds are considered under milch category.

80. True According to the latest livestock census cattle population is decreasing and buffalo population is increasing in India.

81. True Animal and farm waste management through vermin biotechnology is a profitable and eco-friendly activity at dairy farm in present time.

82. True Lactation length in buffalo can be increased through improved management practices.

83. True Reproductive disorder in crossbred cattle and buffalo is the major problem in livestock production in present days.

84. False Pregnancy diagnosis should be done after one month of service through physical palpation of uterine horn in cattle and buffalo.

85. False Colostrum should be fed 6 hrs after the birth of calf in cattle and buffalo.

86. True One milkman can perform milking in morning and evening in 12 buffalo in a day.

87. True About 66% human population of India depends for cooking energy on cow dung.

88. True One bull can produce 80 to100 progenies in a year through natural service.

89. True Average holding of cattle and buffalo in India is 2 to 3 per farmer.

90. True — Loose housing of dairy cattle in Rajasthan is more prevalent and suitable as per climatic conditions.

91. True — Special sets of genes are assigned to control behaviour in animals.

92. True — Monthly milk recording for prediction of milk yield in 300 days is suitable for progeny testing.

Q.2. Multiple Choice Questions :

1. After birth umbilical cord must be treated with:
   a. Potassium permanganate b. Sodium carbonate
   c. Tincture iodine d. Lime water

2. Udder secretion immediately after calving is called:
   a. Calf starter **b. Colostrum**
   c. Skimmed milk d. Yoghurt

3. Milk recording is done on a dairy farm to:
   a. Increase milk yield b. Ensure quality
   c. Help in selection d. Quick sale

4. Teat dipping is done for:
   a. Let down b. More milk production
   c. Prevention of mastitis d. Complete milking

5. Best method of milking dairy animals:
   a. Knuckling b. Wet full hand
   c. Dry full hand d. Stripping

6. Name a disease where carcass of dead animal must be deeply buried with lime powder :
   a. Anthrax b. FMD
   c. Black quarter d. Milk fever

7. Doe is the adult female of:
   a. Pig **b. Goat**
   c. Dog d. Cattle

8. Teaser bull is maintained to:

   a. Protect weak animals b. Mating of buffalo

   c. Detect heat d. Keep herd moving

9. The best age of castration in cattle for preparing bullocks is:

   a. 6 months b. 12 months

   c. 18 months d. 24 months

10. The best method of identification for adult cow is:

    a. Ear notching b. Tattooing

    c. Chemical branding **d. Hot branding**

11. The best age of putting identification marks to adult cow is:

    a. One year b. Two years

    c. Three years d. Four years

12. Number of incisor teeth on the upper jaw of bullock are:

    a. 8 teeth b. 6 teeth

    c. 4 teeth **d. 0 teeth**

13. The bullock of cattle breed famous for swaichal is:

    a. Nagore b. Hariana

    c. Kankrej d. Khillari

14. Sterilization of male calf is known as:

    a. Castration b. Vasectomisation

    c. Spaying d. Hysterectomy

15. A vasectomised male is called:

    a. Steer b. Ox

    c. Teaser d. Bull

16. In a dairy shed the air space per cow should:

    a. 10.5 cubic meter b. 16.5 cubic meter

    c. 22.5 cubic meter d. 28.5 cubic meter

17. One milker can milk:
    a. 6 buffaloes per time
    b. 12 buffaloes per time
    c. 16 buffaloes per time
    d. 20 buffaloes per time

18. The ideal method of hand milking is:
    a. Knuckling
    b. Full hand
    c. Stripping
    d. None of the above

19. Milking pails and system can be sterilized by:
    a. Alkali solution
    b. Acid solution
    c. Chlorine solution
    d. None of the above

20. Microbial culture fed to calves for better digestion and rumen development is called:
    a. Antibiotics
    b. Probiotics
    c. Protected protein
    d. None of the above

21. Famous milch breed of cow in India is:
    a. Tharparker
    b. Hariana
    c. Sahiwal
    d. Kherigarh

22. Flushing is done to increase the:
    a. Ovulation rate only
    b. Conception rate only
    c. Ovulation and conception rate both
    d. None of the above

23. The appropriate age of debudding in cow calves is:
    a. 2 months
    b. 3 months
    c. 10 days
    d. 40 days

24. The appropriate age of castration in cow calves is:
    a. Three months
    b. One year
    c. One and half year
    d. Two years

25. Colostrum is given to newly born calves because it is rich source of:
    a. Protein
    b. Vitamin
    c. Antibodies
    d. All of the above

26. The animal sheds should be located with long axis directed towards:

    a. East to west b. West to east

    c. North to south d. South to north

27. The width of water trough/manger for adult cow is:

    a. 40 cm b. 50 cm

    c. 60 cm **d. 70 cm**

28. Maximum productivity in Indian cattle is achieved by:

    a. 2nd lactation **b. 3rd lactation**

    c. 4th lactation d. 5th lactation

29. Keeping quality of milk can be increased by:

    a. Pasteurization b. Sterilization

    c. boiling **d. All of the above**

30. Sugar of milk is known as:

    a. Glucose b. Sucrose

    c. Lactose d. Fructose

31. Indian breeds crossed with exotic breeds in the All India Coordinated Research Project on cattle were:

    a. Hariana, Gir, Angole

    b. Hariana, Gir, Ongole, Sahiwal

    c. Sindhi, Gir, Tharparkar, Ongole

    d. Hariana, Gir, Ongole, Tharparkar

32. The objective of All India Coordinated Research Project on cattle was to evolve breed or strain of dairy cattle capable of yielding an average of:

    a. 2000 kg of milk b. 3000 kg of milk

    c. 3200 kg of milk d. 3500 kg of milk

33. Latest technology for freezing semen is with:

    a. Solid ice b. Dry ice

    c. Liquid nitrogen d. Combination of a & b

34. Which of the following ingredients will make the ration bulky:
    a. Soyabean meal   b. Ground nut cake
    c. Rice bran   d. Cotton seed cake
35. Correct milking technique is to use:
    a. Wet milking   **b. Dry milking**
    c. Stripping   d. Stroking
36. Optimum dry period for a cow should be:
    a. 90 days   b. 45 days
    c. 75 days   **d. 60 days**
37. The floor space requirement of a down calver (pregnant animal):
    a. 12 x 24 sqm.   **b. 12 x 12 sqm.**
    c. 12 x 36 sqm.   d. 12 x 6 sqm.
38. The wet dry ratio in herd should be:
    a. 75:25   b. 90:10
    c. 40:60   d. 50:50
39. The gestation period of cattle is:
    a. 280 days   b. 310 days
    c. 340 days   d. 210 days
40. Kankrej and Malvi breed of cattle can be classified on the basis of their horn shape:
    a. Lateral horn   **b. Lyre horned**
    c. Long horned   d. Short horned
41. The replacement rate at an organized farm ranges between:
    a. 20-25 %   b. 35-40 %
    c. 50-60 %   d. 100 %
42. The average recorded life span of dairy cattle is:
    a. 10 years   **b. 15-20 years**
    c. 40 years   d. 50 years

43. Most intensive labour operation at farm:

    a. Milking b. Feeding

    c. Watering d. Washing

44. The floor of the milking byre and calf pen should be made up of:

    a. Kanker b. Brick on edge

    c. Concrete cement d. Sand

45. Hectare of land required for ten cows unit dairy farm to maintain fodder supply round the year:

    a. One hectare b. Two hectare

    c. Three hectare d. Four hectare

46. Milking should be completed within:

    a. 5-7 minute b. 30 minute

    c. 60 minute d. 60 second

47. Cattle and buffalo population respectively, in India (million):

    a. 284 & 84 b. 400 & 40

    c. 500 & 50 d. 300 & 75

48. Wallowing is preferred by:

    a. Cattle **b. Buffalo**

    c. Cattle and buffalo d. None of the above

49. The state producing maximum milk:

    a. U.P. b. Bihar

    c. Rajsthan d. Punjab

50. Development strategy followed in breed tracts of pure buffaloes:

    a. Grading up **b. Selective breeding**

    c. Cross breeding d. Inbreeding

51. The optimum group size of dairy cows for loose housing is:

    a. 10-15 b. 20-25

    c. 25-35 d. 45-50

52. Practice of feeding extra concentrate to animals during last quarter of pregnancy is termed as:

    a. Flushing
    b. Wallowing
    c. Grooming
    d. Steaming up

53. Separating neonates from mother and allowing to feeding other than suckling is termed as:

    a. Weaning
    b. Grafting
    c. Rearing
    d. Roughening

54. The floor space requirement of a bull is:

    a. 12 x 24 sq.m.
    b. 12 x 12 sq.m.
    c. 12 x 36 sq.m.
    d. 12 x 6 sq.m.

55. Calving interval is equal to:

    a. Gestation + dry period
    b. Service period + gestation period+ dry period
    c. Lactation length + dry period
    d. None of the above

56. Gestation length of buffalo ranges:

    a. 300-310 days
    b. 275-280 days
    c. 320-400 days
    d. 200-250 days

57. The bull selected initially on the basis of genetic merit should meet the:

    a. Freedom from diseases transmissible through semen
    b. Satisfactory sexual performance
    c. Good semen freezability
    d. All of the above

58. Majority of breeds of cattle in India are:

    a. Dairy breed
    b. Draught breed
    c. Dual breed
    d. All of the above

59. What is not the component of calf starter:

    a. Barley
    b. Ground nut cake
    c. Wheat bran
    d. Avali hay

60. The state which has the highest cow population:

a.	**Uttar Pradesh**	b.	Bihar
c.	Rajsthan	d.	Gujrat

61. Buffalo contributes total milk production of the country (percent):

a.	42 %	b.	47 %
c.	**52 %**	d.	57 %

62. The best dual purpose breed of India is:

a.	Gir	b.	Tharparkar
c.	**Kankrej**	d.	Deoni

63. The guiding factor in cattle development has been the urgent need to increase:

a.	**Milk production**	b.	Draft capacity
c.	Disease resistance	d.	Body weight at calving

64. The slope of the standing space towards the gutter is:

a.	1" in 10	b.	1" in 20'
c.	1" in 30'	**d**	**1" in 40'**

65. The length of the standing space in a dairy byre is:

a.	2.o to 3.0 mt	b.	0.5 to 1.0 mt
c.	**1.5 to 1.7 mt**	d.	3.0 to 4.0 mt

66. The optimum ambient temperature for better comfort to production of dairy cattle should be:

a.	5-7^{0}C	b.	8-12^{0}C
c.	**13-18^{0}C**	d.	30-36^{0}C

67. Gestation length of cattle is:

a.	**284 days**	b.	300 days
c.	310 days	d.	320 days

68. The maintenance requirement of digestible crude protein for an adult buffalo is about:

a. 500 g DCP **b. 300 g DCP**

c. 200 g DCP d. 100 g DCP

69. The water requirement of a lactating cow weighing 500 kg producing 15 kg of milk per day is:

a. 25 lit. b. 45 lit.

c. 70 lit. d. 35 lit.

70. The age (week) at which the calf starter is generally introduced for feeding of calf:

a. 2nd b. 3rd

c. 4th d. 5th

71. Place of habitation in buffaloes is called a:

a. Byre b. Pen

c. Stable d. Sty

72. Artificial insemination has been accepted as the best method of breeding because:

a. Less cost is involved in processing semen

b. Want of proven superior quality sire

c. Checking brucellosis only

d. None of the above

73. Which one of the Indian cattle breeds is used for grading up of non descriptive cattle in Uttarakhand:

a. Hariana **b. Red Sindhi**

c. Tharparkar d. Gir

74. Which one of the optimum culling rate should be followed at dairy farm for improvement:

a. 10-15% **b. 20-25%**

c. 30-35% d. 40-45%

75. On a dairy farm, (240 milking cows) the number of livestock attendants required for feeding, washing and milking would be:

a. 10-12 | **b. 20-24**
c. 30-34 | d. 40-42

76. All India Key Village Scheme was launched to meet the shortage of:

a. Bulls | b. Milk
c. Fodder | d. Cows

77. The guiding factor in cattle and buffalo breeding project has been urgent need to increase:

a. Milk production | b. Draught capacity
c. Disease resistance | d. Body weight at calving

78. Which one of the following buffalo breed is used on a large scale for grading up of non descriptive buffalo:

a. Bhadawari | b. Nili Ravi
c. Murrah | d. Surti

79. Which one of the following state has maximum cattle and buffalo population:

a. Bihar | b. Rajasthan
c. U.P. | d. Gujarat

80. Which one of the following is the best draught cattle breed:

a. Ongole | b. Hariana
c. Nagori | d. Tharparkar

81. Which one of the following is the optimum age of semen collection to crossbred cattle:

a. 10-12 months | **b. 18-20 months**
c. 22-24 months | d. 26-28 months

82. Which one of the following percentage is the cost of production of feeding of livestock:

a. 50 | b. 60
c. 70 | d. 80

83. Colostrum is not rich in one following milk constituents:

a. Casein
b. Albumin
c. Immunoglobulin
d. Fat

84. Which one of the following disease had been eradicated from cattle in India.

a. Food and mouth disease
b. Hemorrhagic septicemia
c. Rinderpest
d. Black quarter

85. Which one of the following management practices will contribute to enhance milk productivity in dairy animals:

a. Breeding
b. Feeding
c. Health care
d. All of the above

86. Crystoscope developed by IVRI is used to detect:

a. Harmful pathogen in semen
b. Appropriate time for insemination
c. Adulteration in milk
d. All of the above

87. Which one of the effective technology and methodology for genetic improvement is used in dairy cattle and buffalo:

a. Grading up
b. Crossbreeding
c. Progeny testing and sire evaluation
d. Pedigree selection

88. Which one of the following organizations has evolved Frieswal crossbred cattle strain:

a. NDDB Anand
b. NDRI Karnal
c. 45 military farms of India and project directorate on cattle
d. Kerala livestock development board

Q.3. Fill up the Blanks :

1. Best breed of buffalo is ***Murrah.***
2. Black gold of India is ***Murrah*.**
3. Highest milk fat is found in ***Bhadawari*** buffalo.
4. India possesses around ***20*** percent of bovine population of the world.
5. India produces around ***10*** percent milk of world.
6. DM requirement per 100 kg BW is ***2.5 kg.***
7. Water requirement per litre of milk is ***4 litres.***
8. Best Indian milch breed of cow is ***Sahiwal.***
9. Best age for weaning of calf is at ***birth.***
10. Best housing system is ***loose.***
11. Best method of hand milking is ***dry hand/full hand.***
12. One milker is required for milking ***14*** dairy animals
13. Operation flood started in the year ***1970.***
14. Best age for debudding a calf is ***7-10 days.***
15. Best time for feeding colostrum after birth is ***within 2hrs. of birth.***
16. Gir cattle have ***long curled*** ears.
17. In unified score card method of judging dairy cows ***20*** marks are allotted for body capacity.
18. The bypass protein is ***not*** synthesized by rumen micro flora.
19. The milk fat percent is ***negatively*** associated with milk yield.
20. Gujarat has three distinct breeds of buffalo namely ***Jaffarabadi, Surti and Mehsana*.**
21. India has ***26*** breeds of cattle and ***8 breeds*** of buffalo.
22. The feeding of pregnant females with an extra ration during last stage of pregnancy is known as ***steaming up*.**
23. The process by which reproductive organs of a female return back to their original position and size after calving is called ***involution*.**
24. To improve the dairy herd the rate of culling annually should be ***20-25*** percent.

25. Cows are generally rebred at ***60-90*** days after calving.
26. ***Hot branding*** is the best method of identification of large ruminants under field conditions.
27. In stall housing one cow require space measuring ***1.5*** meter in length and ***1.2*** meter in width.
28. The optimum ambient temperature for better comfort and production of cattle should be ***13-18ºC.***
29. Lay out of the farm is intended to show ***size, number and location.***
30. The buffaloes in India may be improved through ***selective breeding.***
31. Breeds used under All India Coordinated Research Project on buffalo are ***Murrah and Surti.***
32. Majority of breeds of cattle in India are ***draught*** breed.
33. Buffalo breed famous for regular breeding is ***Surti***
34. Scientific name of Indian buffalo is ***Bubalus bubalis.***
35. Rectal temperature under normal physiological condition in cattle is ***101.5±0.5ºF.***
36. The average estrus period in buffalo is ***18-24 hrs.***
37. Feeding of dairy cattle costs ***70%*** age of total cost of milk production.
38. Number of incisors present in the upper jaw of cow is ***zero.***
39. Normally placenta is expelled within ***10-12 hrs***. after calving.
40. Recommended body weight of a heifer at the time of first breeding should be approximately ***280-300*** kg.
41. The right age for brucellosis vaccination is ***3-6 months.***
42. KVS stands for ***key village scheme.***
43. The optimum group size of cow for loose housing system should be ***30-40.***
44. In bull, nose ring should be applied by the age of ***one year.***
45. Lola is a breed of ***Sahiwal.***
46. First military dairy farm was started at ***Allahabad.***
47. In a lactating cow, milk production reaches the peak approximately ***two months*** after calving.

48. The cattle population in India is about ***195*** million.
49. Three exotic cattle breed involved in All India Coordinated Research Project on cattle are ***Holstein Friesian, Brown Swiss and Jersey.***
50. Indian buffaloes constitute ***52*** percent of the total world buffalo population.
51. To remove or prevent growth of horn buds in heifer is called ***disbudding.***
52. For dairy cattle, broadly two types of livestock houses are made namely ***loose*** and ***close.***
53. Slope of the drain should be ***1 in 40.***
54. Important climatic elements which influence the livestock production are ***temperature, humidity and rainfall.***
55. In loose housing system the length of feeding trough should be ***1 to 1.2*** meter per cow.
56. Feed stuff high in crude fibre and low in digestible nutrients is known as ***roughage.***
57. The annual stock replacement rate at a large diary farm should be ***15 to 20*** percent.
58. Milking cows require ***45-70*** litres of water for drinking per day.
59. Chewing the cud is called the process of ***rumination.***
60. The calf starter should have about ***20*** percent crude protein and not more than ***5*** percent fibre.
61. An insufficient supply of energy in the ration ***retards*** the growth and ***delay*** puberty.
62. If the cow is frightened, angered or ill treated ***let down*** of milk will not occur and very little milk can be harvested.
63. Indian breeds used under All India Coordinated Research Project on cattle are ***Hariana, Ongole and Gir.***
64. Three common methods of hand milking are ***stripping, full hand method and stroking.***
65. ***KOH/NaOH*** used in chemical dehorning of calves.
66. The system in which animals are tied for most of the time is called ***closed housing*** system.

67. Buffaloes like to ***wallowing*** in ponds, canals when environmental temperature is high.

68. In a dairy herd the ideal proportion of milk and dry cows should be ***75:25.***

69. Separation of neonates from mother so that they can no longer suckle is called ***weaning.***

70. ***Cement concrete*** flooring is suitable for calf pens.

71. In machine milking milk is taken out from the udder by use of a ***vacuum*** in side the milk machine inflation.

72. The two most practical tests used for detecting mastitis are the ***strip cup test*** and ***California mastitis test.***

73. The rumen of a new born calf becomes functional at the age of ***6 to 7*** week under usual farm condition.

74. ***Massage of udder*** should be practiced before commencement of actual milking operation.

75. Female bovine before its first calf is known as ***heifer.***

76. ***Murrah and Nili Ravi*** have the highest milk production potential followed by Surti, Jaffarabadi, Mehsana and bhadawari.

77. Bloody mucus from vagina is an indicator of ***infection in uterus.***

78. Conception of dairy cow and buffalo must occur within ***90*** days of post partum.

79. ***Pedigree history sheet*** is one of the important records of dairy animals which provide productive reproductive traits and pedigree information.

80. Branding involves smearing a number on the skin of an animal with ***hot iron and chemical.***

81. The average quantity of dung excreted by Indian cow, buffalo and crossbred cattle per day is ***10kg, 15kg and 20kg*** respectively.

82. The house for accommodation of advance pregnant cow is known as ***calving pen.***

83. Milch cows and buffaloes should be dried off after about ***305*** days of lactation.

84. In tropical climate ***loose*** housing system may relieve the crossbred cows from heat stress.

85. ***Earthworms*** are used in transformation of animal dung and dairy farm waste into high quality animal protein.

86. Comfortable environment temperature for dairy cattle and buffalo is ***20-30°F.***

87. Preferable ***milch*** cows shed should be located around milking byre and ***non pregnant*** cows around A.I. shed.

88. A milkman should perform milking of ***40-45*** dairy cows in a day by using milking machine.

89. Milk price is fixed based on ***fat and S.N.F.*** constituents of milk by State Cooperative Dairy Federation.

90. Milking in dairy cattle by machine is preferred only in those animals who give more than ***10*** kg milk yield per day.